The Best of
Alternative…from
Alternative's Best

The Best of Alternative...from Alternative's Best

✦

Views of America's Top Alternative Physicians

by Dee Woods

iUniverse, Inc.

New York Lincoln Shanghai

The Best of Alternative...from Alternative's Best
Views of America's Top Alternative Physicians

iUniverse books may be ordered through booksellers or by contacting:

iUniverse
2021 Pine Lake Road, Suite 100
Lincoln, NE 68512
www.iuniverse.com
1-800-Authors (1-800-288-4677)

The information in this book is not meant to diagnose or treat any disorder. It is a compilation of views and research of the nation's top alternative physicians. The information should be shared with your health care professional.

This book is meant to provide readers with the latest information and research available in the form of alternative and integrative newsletters and web sites. All newsletter resources are listed in the back of this book under "Resources" to enable readers to have access to the research of these fine health professionals.

ISBN-13: 978-0-595-38162-3 (pbk)
ISBN-13: 978-0-595-82530-1 (ebk)
ISBN-10: 0-595-38162-6 (pbk)
ISBN-10: 0-595-82530-3 (ebk)

Printed in the United States of America

To three precious miracles, our triplet grandsons, Carlos, Dario and Emilio

Contents

Introduction

The emergency room was exceptionally quiet that dreary February morning. I was somewhat numb but thankfully, I learned the stroke my husband suffered was mild; however, what would follow, in the form of "treatment" over the next 30 days would prove as devastating as the stroke itself.

Initially my husband was stabilized and placed on medication for high blood pressure. The wise neurologist then decided to treat him with baby aspirin and Atenolol blood pressure medication. She wanted to maintain that regime until it could be determined exactly what caused his stroke. "Conservative treatment," she said. He was doing so well and he appeared to be on the road to recovery, but he needed a week or two of physical therapy for his affected right side. The news sounded good, and he was in excellent spirits but that would soon change once he was transferred to another hospital for two weeks of physical therapy.

It was at that hospital I made two major discoveries: the first being that I was "invisible." The second, learning that many conventional doctors live by the sword of pharmaceuticals.

"Aggressive treatment" the new doctor said. "He had a stroke, he needs aggressive treatment." Apparently the new doctor was of the opinion strokes require extraordinary pharmacuetical intervention, even when the patient was doing quite well on conservative treatment. So, new medications were piled on daily. The new doctor was never around long enough to notice that with each new medication my husband began losing ground. I told the doctor. But I'm not a doctor so my observation didn't count.

My husband became extremely ill from the heparin, developed a small superficial blood clot in the calf and then went on to be prescribed numerous other medications—blood thinners, cholesterol medications, triglyceride medication, and additional blood pressure pills.

I helplessly watched his condition deteriorate. Finally, from very classic symptoms they should have observed, it was clear to me that he was bleeding internally. I informed them of what was happening. They wryly smiled and assured me all was well because his blood tests from that morning were fine. But this was afternoon and he began slipping away. I pled with them to do something. They ignored me. He continued to slip as I continued to plead. I felt like the mythological figure, Cassandra. No one would believe me.

Finally, late that evening, his hemoglobin plummeted to 7.4 (he entered the facility with a count of 15). He went into shock and his kidneys failed. Only then did doctors decide he needed blood and plasma. They sheepishly avoided me never bothering to acknowledge my observations had been correct and, indeed, he had been bleeding internally. He then had endoscopic surgery to stop the bleed and thankfully, his kidney function returned. I was thankful to God he survived, but the effects of his stroke were exacerbated by the trauma to his system. He could now barely move.

They stabilized him and informed me he would need another two to three weeks "treatment" in the hospital. Hah! As my mother would say, "In a pig's eye!"

Still stunned by the ordeal and more than slightly angry at their unwillingness to consider my observations, I advised them I was bringing him home immediately. I was petrified because I didn't know exactly how I would be able to care for him. He was quite disabled and required constant attention.

The next two years were somewhat grueling. We participated in courses of physical therapy, diet and exercise. He is now doing somewhat better but not as well as he would have had he not suffered that unnecessary setback.

Medical arrogance and disregard for familial observations are up there along with the notion there is a pill for every ill. I felt a need to research and write about integrative approaches to healing as well as the dangers of some FDA approved medications.

American medicine is in trouble. Many doctors are content in treating and masking symptoms rather than in taking the time to seek and treat the causes of illness.

This book is for average people who might be interested in integrative and alternative views and would like to know more about what integrative and alternative physicians believe. Resources and addresses of some of the country's top alternative health professionals are listed in the back of the book.

Acknowledgements

"Friends are angels who lift us to our feet when our wings have trouble remembering how to fly." ~ *Author Unknown* ~

First, I would like to thank my sister, Diane who has been my most ardent cheerleader and supporter. Diane's constant urgings and assistance gave me the courage to put forth the effort and I thank her for being my strongest ally and such a wonderful friend.

My husband and my sons, Paul and Brent have been equally supportive. Each of them has assisted me in completing the book.

My friend Sue Murawski was the first to be there after my husband's stroke—lending her quiet strength, looking out for me and helping me adjust to a dramatically changed life. Jackie and Greg Spacek are my old friends who also served as anchors during and after my husband's stroke. They have always been great friends.

I would also like to thank a special friend, Camille "Kami" Krecioch, graphic designer, for her creative talents in designing my book cover. I especially appreciate the time Kami has devoted to me and my efforts in completing this book. Her exceptional sense of humor has served to help lighten the load along the way.

Then there's another friend, Paul Dakuras who organized my chaotic office—albeit with a bit of "constructive" criticism. He enabled me to begin preparing the content for the book by assuring I could easily access my information—as well as locate my computer! Most of all, I am thankful for his friendship and moral support.

Shortly after my husband's stroke, local editor of The Reporter Newspaper, Jack Murray, called to see how I was doing. "Big mistake," I said. I "unloaded" my frustrations on Jack's shoulders as he listened with great compassion. It was during that conversation, Jack reminded me of my earlier desires to write an alternative health column and it was during that conversation I decided to take him up on the offer he extended that day.

I thank Charles Richards, publisher of the Reporter/Regional newspapers who has also supported my efforts and graciously offered his help. Then there's Jason Maholy, my current editor. I appreciate his professional opinions as well as his editing and copyediting. I am thankful for his input on my composition as well as on the content of my articles. He is wonderful to work with.

My old friend, Mike Bates has provided many years of friendship and I'm glad he's there when I need advice.

Very special thanks to Steve and Annette Cardamone for being the first to offer me a spot at their establishment, Eagle Textbooks, for the sale of my book upon publication.

Dee Woods can be reached at deewoods@comcast.net

ACETAMINOPHEN: WATCH FOR LIVER DAMAGE

At the first sign of a headache or when that nagging back pain strikes, many people take a Tylenol without a second thought. We have been conditioned to use acetaminophen and no one bothered telling us it can be dangerous to the liver over time or when over-used.

The liver performs more than 400 separate daily functions, each devoted to transforming food into nutrients and storing nutrients. It also eliminates the daily toxins we never realized we ingested throughout the day. It is important to refrain from practices that damage the liver, such as abusive drinking, and it is important to avoid overloading the liver with products that can put a stress on it, such as acetaminophen.

In the most recent November 2002 Public Citizen newsletter it was reported that in l999 there were 108,000 calls to Poison Control Centers and an average of 56,500 emergency room visits, 26,000 hospital confinements and an average of 458 deaths associated with taking acetaminophen (the active ingredient in Tylenol). They state most were unintentional overdoses.

How does an overdose occur?

One of the reasons for overdose is that patients take several over-the-counter painkillers not realizing each individual product they are taking may contain acetaminophen. Over 100 million people a year take acetaminophen. The figure is probably a great deal larger since there are about 200 pain medications that contain acetaminophen. Additionally, many over-the-counter and prescribed medications for other non-pain related medical conditions have a negative effect on the liver. Cumulative effect can pose a problem.

Babies and acetaminophen

Another problem is associated with using the liquid form for babies. Unfortunately, some parents simply use teaspoonfuls instead of the droppers that come with the product. Most parents are unaware Tylenol suspension contains as much as 1/3 more of the drug per milliliter as acetaminophen drops, according to the folks at Public Citizen. This misunderstanding can cause unintentional overdose, according to the organization. Healthy livers can readily metabolize small amounts of Acetaminophen. We run into trouble when the liver must process a large increase in dosage.

What's good for the liver?

The authors of Health Science newsletter state, N-acetylcysteine (NAC) an amino acid, is an antidote for acetaminophen poisoning especially when used within 8 hours of the overdose. It stimulates production of glutathione, a most potent antioxidant enzyme. "This ability to infuse the liver with antioxidants, coupled with excellent anti-inflammatory properties, makes NAC an effective liver crisis treatment. Studies have shown that NAC treatments may significantly decrease the chance of mortality in patients suffering from acute liver damage," claim the authors of Health Science Institute.

They also suggest that milk thistle has been shown to stimulate the production of new liver cells, and is often used to help protect the liver from alcohol damage and to treat liver diseases. "Turmeric root, like NAC, is reputed to have powerful antioxidant and anti-inflammatory effects that promote healthy liver function. And burdock helps to stimulate the liver's ability to purify the blood" according to the publication.

Alpha Lipoic acid, selenium and Vitamins C and E are also good antioxidants for the liver as well as B-vitamins, zinc and lecithin.

A simple aid to the liver is to eat more raw fruits and vegetables that will benefit the entire system.

Alternatives?

"Fortunately there are alternatives to acetaminophen in treating headache, fever, muscle aches, menstrual cramps and toothaches. For instance, the herb white willow is an anti-inflammatory pain reliever that has compounds similar to aspirin. In fact, white willow salicylic acid is the parent compound of aspirin (acetylsalicylic acid). Salicylic acid, however, has the benefit of being less abrasive to the stomach and intestine. And a study recently published in the Journal, *Rheumatology* showed an extract of willow tree bark to be as effective as a prescription drug in the treatment of lower back pain," according to the folks at Health Science

Institute. Studies have shown the herb, feverfew to be effective for migraines as well.

Acetaminophen provides some needed relief and assistance when absolutely needed, but be careful when consuming large amounts for extensive periods of time or when taking other medications along with the acetaminophen. Check to see what other more natural means can be used to fend off that headache without putting your liver on the line.

You may also be interested to know that according to Dr. Joseph Mercola's web site data, studies have found that cold remedies, Tylenol, etc. cause healing time to take longer. University of Maryland-Baltimore Schools of Pharmacy and Medicine showed that drug takers suffer flu symptoms for an average 3.5 days longer than those who went untreated. Chickenpox sufferers treated with acetaminophen required more time for sores to heal.

ACIDOPHILUS (PROBIOTICS) WHEN USING ANTIBIOTICS

The last time your doctor prescribed antibiotics for a health condition, did he/she also prescribe probiotics? If your doctor suggested supplementing with probiotics, you are fortunate.

We are all familiar with the word "antibiotic" however; few are familiar with the word "probiotic" which has an equally important function in promoting our body's natural immunity. "Probiotics" is from the Greek "for life". Acidophilus is the most common form of good bacteria.

Antibiotics destroy our good bacteria

Antibiotics can be effective in killing bad bacteria; unfortunately, antibiotics are unable to distinguish between good bacteria necessary for proper digestion and bad bacteria that harm our bodies. Antibiotics kill both the good and bad bacteria. They create a type of "collateral damage" that wipes out our friendly flora within the intestines, while attacking dangerous bacteria. Over the years, patients have been prescribed antibiotics without the necessary probiotics to mitigate the damage caused by the antibiotics.

Friendly bacteria—good soldiers

Consider the friendly bacteria in your intestines as good soldiers creating balance and protecting your system from dangerous outside forces such as those forces that create yeast overgrowth. Women especially, are subject to yeast infections after a course of antibiotics, hence, the need to supplement with probiotics. Those who are subject to yeast infections without antibiotics may also do well to supplement with probiotics. Some probiotics are found in some yogurts and in buttermilk. They can also be found in health food stores in the refrigerated section.

Probiotics provide many necessary functions

Our friendly soldiers have been greatly overlooked and underrated over the years and only recently is their essential function to our overall good health being recognized and appreciated. Why? Because we have learned our friendly bacteria help to:

- assist us in the absorption of minerals and vitamins and help improve our digestion.

- protect and improve immune function and increase the absorption of calcium.

- help produce our "B" vitamins.

- assist in controlling yeast in the system.

- Protect us against other harmful bacteria and fungus.

As you can see, our friendly soldiers have numerous essential functions that work throughout our entire systems; yet, many physicians have failed to recognize the importance of replacing them, especially after prescribing antibiotics.

Poor eating habits also destroy friendly bacteria

Many patients are treated with antacids and medications for persistent gas and intestinal discomfort, when in fact; replacing the friendly bacteria may be of greater long-term assistance. Because our friendly bacteria have become sparse due to antibiotic usage and poor eating habits over the years, the good bacteria cannot provide adequate digestive function. The absence of probiotics can result in bloating, gas, diarrhea/constipation, skin conditions as well as other immune disorders.

If you decide to try probiotics, do not expect immediate results. It may take a few months of usage to see major improvement in your symptoms and to build up your army of friendly bacteria, but stick with it. Remember, it took many years of antibiotic usage and poor eating habits to bring us to these points of discomfort, so let's have patience in our quest to restore healthy intestines and a healthy immune system. It's worth the effort.

AGING GRACEFULLY? NOT YET! LET'S TALK ANTI-AGING

It's not about aging gracefully, it's about aging and remaining as healthy as possible in order to keep those golden years from turning rusty. Over the last few years, I have found a number of useful tools aside from the usual "be happy, limit calories and exercise" routine. I believe in all of those suggestions but there's a great deal more to the aging process.

We have learned of the benefits of Coenzyme Q10 for heart health and energy levels, but it also appears to act as an anti-aging tool. Coenzyme Q10 optimizes mitochondrial function according to Dale Kiefer who writes about anti-aging in the February 2005 issue of *Life Extension Magazine*.

In many cases, stress creates conditions within our bodies that throw our systems out of whack. Stress is devastating to our overall health. It is a certain precursor to aging. It's that simple.

On the stress front, another mitochondrial optimizer written of in the same issue helps fight the effects of stress. The stress fighter is a plant known as rhodiola rosea. I was aware this particular plant was useful for fighting stress-related activities; however, it appears to do much more than originally believed. According to the author, rhodiola helps in creating a balance in the entire body. It is known as an "adaptogen" which means it assists in bringing the system into a state of homeostasis (balance) by secondarily helping the body increase resistance to chemical, physical and biological assaults. Adaptogens are believed to facilitate the body in recovering both after exercise and illness. Russian athletes, cosmonauts and elderly politicians have used Rhodiola since its discovery in 1969. It was approved for use in Sweden in 1975.

A number of small studies have shown it to optimize brain serotonin and dopamine levels while having a positive influence on beta-endorphins, which give us that sense of "well-being." The unfortunate side of this plant extract is that it is not recommended for treatment of bipolar disorders.

Rhodiola is also helpful in preventing the aging process according to the article in *Life Extension Magazine*. It has been shown to enhance endurance exercise capacity as it optimizes the mitochondrial health of each cell. In early animal studies it has been shown to slow tumor growth as well as metastases. Another of the benefits of rhodiola is that it appears to enhance thyroid function. An under active thyroid can sometimes create weight gain and has been shown to have a negative psychological impact. Since rhodiola is known to increase energy levels and enhance physical endurance, weight loss may naturally be another unsung benefit of rhodiola. Remember also, the thyroid has a great deal to do with both physical and mental health.

Rhodiola appears to have many useful functions in the anti-aging arena, but it should be used with the assistance of your physician so that the dosage can be adjusted up or down. The article explains smaller doses are used for those with anxiety disorders while the larger dosage appears to help with depression. It is also not recommended for constant use but should be discontinued after a few weeks before restarting again.

Additionally, from the studies I've seen, Siberian rhodiola rosea is more effective than plants from any other region of the world. It appears to have more of the constituents that work together to enhance the mitochondria. The studies are encouraging and the fact that there are multiple medical and psychological benefits to this plant should send a message to the conventional medical community. Why not insist on larger studies instead of creating new chemicals that result in liver stress and other negative side effects for treating psychological and physical disorders.

The *Life Extension* article explains, "Mitochondria create energy in the form of ATP (adenosine triphosphate)—a molecule that humans literally could not live without." The explanation becomes very technical and explains how our mitochondria die off, many times in premature fashion, hastening the aging process.

An amino acid known as L-carnitine is another of those properties that help improve mitochondrial function systemically. The amino acid was first isolated from meat "carnus" in 1905; hence the word, "carnitine" was coined. L-Carnitine is synthesized in the liver and kidneys where it must be transported to other tissues, especially those that utilize fatty acids as fuels. Our hearts, skeleton and body muscle all require fatty acids to maintain proper function. L-carnitine helps by creating energy to the mitochrondria for metabolism.

In fact, an article that appeared in Pediatric Magazine in 2000 reported the importance of L-carnitine for treatment in children with cardiomyopathy. It appears to be a very important supplement in the treatment of childhood heart disease. Interesting. It's not a medication, yet it is suggested for use among children with heart disease. That alone should speak volumes about the efficacy of L-carnitine for mitochondrial health in adults.

L-Carnitine in the form of acetyl L-carnitine arginyl amide (a metabolite of L-carnitine), was shown in studies to stimulate brain cells, "…prompting them to grow new connections to other neurons." according *to Life Extension* magazine. The LEF article goes on to explain the studies on brain protective qualities of L-carnitine and its metabolites. In one study, aging rats showed drastic improvement in age-related brain lipid composition as well as having increased energy levels when supplemented with L-carnitine. The studies indicate the need for such supplementation with L-carnitine among the older population. That could explain why cardiologist, Stephen Sinatra has added L-carnitine to his coenzyme Ql0 supplements. He believes the two work synergistically to enhance both heart health and energy levels. Dr. Joseph Mercola goes so far as to say L-carnitine should always be used as "part of routine care for congestive heart failure."

An exciting notation *in Life Extension* Foundation Magazine states, "Acetyl-L-carnitine arginate's ability to stimulate new growth by neurons is extraordinarily significant. Brain nerve cells, unlike other cells in the body are generally incapable of repairing themselves." They go on to explain how important this is to the treatment of neuronal degenerative diseases such as Parkinson's and Alzheimer's. These are all of the latest studies and many physicians may not even be aware of the findings to date. It's important that we learn of these studies and if our physicians are unaware of the results, we can suggest they research the latest available information on such topics.

There is no one magic pill, however, when we assure adequate intake of the necessary amino acids, fatty acids, herbs and vitamins, we give our bodies a better chance at dealing with today's stresses and fighting off the aging process.

For further information on L-carnitine you may be interested in a book by Robert Crayhorn: "The Carnitine Miracle."

We have only touched on a few of the basics involved in anti-aging, but those I covered are major factors according to the authors of *Life Extension Foundation* magazine. There are many components to fighting the aging process. Extending and enhancing mitochondrial health is only a beginning.

Another approach written of is enabling the body to fight the glycation process. Glycation is what happens when protein chemically bonds or cross-links with sugar molecules. This process begins the journey that leads us to wrinkles, and inflexibility of skin and organs. According to "Life Extension" magazine, advanced glycation is what leads to triggering inflammatory reactions as well as premature aging.

So what helps aside from avoiding the sugar bowl? Carnosine—according to the magazine. Carnosine consists of two linked amino acids known as "dipep-tides." Carnosine has been shown to stop advanced glycation and even to reverse the damage of advanced glycation. The authors state, "Glycation occurs when proteins or DNA molecules chemically bond, or cross-link, with sugar molecules. Eventually the sugars are further modified, forming advanced glycation end prod-ucts that ultimately cross-link with adjacent proteins, rendering tissue increas-ingly stiff and inflexible." The authors further go on to explain the reaction to glycation in the laboratory: "For instance, when added to living cells growing in culture, carnosine extend the cells' life span. When added to decrepit aged cells it rejuvenates them."

Carnosine not only possesses antioxidant capacity but it "appears to reverse glycation by directly reacting with carbonyl groups that consist of an oxygen atom joined by a double bond with a carbon atom. Alone, these chemical entities are called carbon monoxide." They go on to explain that carbon monoxide attaches to proteins, causing the ultimate damage that causes aging. Carnosine appears to alter defective proteins and allow the body to eliminate them through the cellular process. The effects of this activity stop advanced glycation; hence, less cellular damage to cause aging and disease.

Another assistant is R-lipoic acid. I wrote of Dr. Burt Berkson's use of lipoic acid for fighting liver damage and hepatitis C, but it appears to have many more significant qualities in the aging process. The "R" form of lipoic acid appears to be more potent and when researchers added it to acetyl-L-carnitine, it had even greater antioxidant activity. A study conducted at the National Cancer Institute in Italy, indicated that lipoic acid is showing great promise with neurological dis-orders such as multiple sclerosis.

Life Extension magazine is one of my favorites because they always note and cite individual studies and lists those studies at the end of each article. This par-ticular article on anti-aging has 90 cites.

So when we think of those things that fight the aging process, coenzyme Q10 is at the top of the list with L-carnitine, carnosine and R-lipoic acid. Of course, there are many other variables involved in planning an anti-aging strategy, but by becoming informed about some of the major factors, we can be a step ahead of convention.

Talk with your physician about the studies and see if he/she is willing to learn more in order to help you as a patient.

ALZHEIMER'S DISEASE: VIEWS FROM THE ALTERNATIVE COMMUNITY

Are heavy metals a factor?

One word certain to send shivers down the spines of many Americans is "Alzheimer's." Numerous researchers and physicians are attempting to find causes of Alzheimer's. There are serious early clues that will probably not be addressed for years to come.

Brain impairment has many causes—among them—trauma, tumor, drugs, environmental pollutants, medications and even something as simple as dehydration—not drinking enough good water.

Robert Jay Rowen, M.D., author of *Second Opinion*, newsletter, has some interesting views on what he and other alternative physicians believe contributes to causes of Alzheimer's. Because he is not alone in his views, and his suggestions are logical and healthful regardless, they are worth repeating.

Rowen believes ingestion and bodily application of aluminum containing products, fluoride, mercury, high homocysteine levels and deficiencies of various nutrients, all contribute to the increase in Alzheimer's disease. He also believes another cause that may affect brain deterioration is misdiagnosing a case of hypothyroidism (low thyroid production).

Aluminum connection

Rowen noted that among Alzheimer's patients there are toxic metals within the brain. Aluminum is one of those metals. He cites an April 1996 report in the British medical journal, The Lancet, implicating aluminum as a toxin found in the brains of Alzheimer's patients and prolonged aluminum ingestion as a cause of the development of Alzheimer's. We are exposed to tremendous amounts of aluminum. Aluminum is used in cooking utensils, cans, anti-perspirants, tap water (used to clarify and remove acids from water), toothpaste, some baking preparations and even some antacids. Rowen cites Australian authorities and asks the question, "Why has Australia's biggest city, Sydney, weaned its citizens off aluminum treated water due to concerns about the link between aluminum and Alzheimer's?" He suggests we read labels on everything we ingest, cook with or apply to our bodies including anti-perspirants and deodorants containing aluminum. He notes that most American city water systems add aluminum, fluoride and chlorine to the tap water. He suggests these toxins be removed before drinking the water. Since aluminum is not a nutrient and is highly toxic, why not avoid ingestion or absorption as much as possible?

Missing Hypothyroidism

Rowen explains that low thyroid function can cause conditions that appear as Alzheimer's. Again, he cites a report in Discover magazine, February 1988. Dr. Oliver Sacks of Albert Einstein College of Medicine reported that several cases diagnosed as Alzheimer's, were, in fact, cases of undiagnosed hypothyroidism. Dr. Rowen feels that these missed diagnoses may be more prevalent than most realize. He feels that nursing homes and private hospitals may well have more than a few cases of hypothyroidism diagnosed as Alzheimer's or senility.

Fluoride connection

Rowen is also among those who feel that the fluoride in tap water causes the body to absorb more aluminum as well as negatively affect the brain and bones. He cites a Chinese study that found that a "fluoride dose of only three to 11 parts per million could affect the nervous system directly, long before the effects of skeletal fluorosis (a bone disease caused by fluoride) became apparent." He noted that many toothpastes contain 1,000 to 1,5000 parts per million of fluoride and users, especially children, should be warned not to swallow any of the paste. Refrain from soft drinks in aluminum cans.

What's good for the brain?

Aside from avoiding the above toxic metals, there are things you can do to help your entire system. It is suggested we start by drinking plenty of good water, eat foods that supply choline, an essential brain nutrient that is contained in eggs, lettuce, cauliflower, steak and oranges. Artichoke and Brazil nuts are also great. Rowen states that anise, sage and saffron are good herbs to use when preparing foods. He states that B-vitamins, especially folic acid, which helps eliminate homocysteine, are very essential as well.

Alzheimer's and Modified Citrus Pectin (MCP) Is Nan Kathryn Fuchs on to something?

Recently, researcher, Nan Kathryn Fuchs, PhD, wrote of her interesting observation regarding possible causes of Alzheimer's disease. She had been reading an article in the February 15, 2003 issue of Lancet, a British medical journal, which suggested a process known as angiogenesis (development of blood vessels) caused progression of Alzheimer's disease. The article suggests that blocking angiogenesis may be the key to halting such progression.

Fuchs was astonished upon reading the report, since she was in the process of writing a booklet on a substance used to fight cancer and heart disease using a product that stopped angiogenesis. The substance in question, modified citrus pectin (MCP), also accomplished these goals through its anti-angiogenesis properties. Angiogenesis is also the process by which cancer tumors reproduce. Angiogenesis feeds tumors by creating new blood vessels that nourish tumors. Fuchs was excited about the Lancet article because she felt her own research might also have new and useful application in halting Alzheimer's disease as well.

What is modified citrus pectin?

Regular citrus pectin is a soluble fiber found in citrus fruits. It is used in bulking agents to relieve constipation and to protect against colon cancer. It is a fiber that cannot penetrate the intestinal walls; however, it does perform a scrubbing action to cleanse the colon. When citrus pectin is modified it is broken down into smaller more uniform molecules that allows it to penetrate the intestinal walls and enter the blood stream to cleanse the entire system. The end product of this alteration of pectin molecules is known as modified citrus pectin. MCP also has unique properties that enable it to chelate (bind to) heavy metals as well as disabling cancer cells, according to Fuchs. She states that MCP inhibits cancer cells from multiplying by creating an anti-angiogenesis process. It halts the formation of blood vessels needed to feed cancer. Fuchs feels she has discovered yet, another use for MCP in fighting Alzheimer's if indeed, the Lancet article is correct.

According to Fuchs, cancer cells are social creatures that must attach themselves to one another. "MCP attaches itself to cancer cells so they can't attach themselves to one another. MCP also stops new blood vessels from forming, cutting off their food supply. Without food, cancer cells starve to death."

It is believed that the actual angiogenesis process is created by inflammation. An inflamed area triggers the formation of new blood vessels, according to Fuchs, which in turn, causes tumor growth. In the case of Alzheimer's, Fuchs says, "Inflammation triggers the formation of new blood vessels and these new blood vessels cause the deposit of plaque and the secretion of a toxin that kills brain cells."

Another study on the application of modified citrus pectin is presently being conducted by California physician Isaac Eliaz, M.D. He is testing MCP as a chelating (bind to) agent in the removal of heavy metals. His preliminary studies have found that those patients given 3 grams of MCP taken 3 times a day are excreting higher urinary levels of heavy metals.

Fuchs closes in saying, "The best part about taking MCP for brain deterioration is that it's working to stop cancer cells from forming tumors and preventing heart disease at the same time that it's stopping Alzheimer's." One of the more common threads about using any naturally occurring food substance is that it generally serves to protect the body in an overall sense.

Dr. Fuchs reports the studies conducted on MCP, were all conducted using one particular form of modified citrus pectin. It is called PectaSol and is available from EcoNugenics at 800-308-5518, Life Extension Foundation 800-544-4440 and Longevity Science 800-993-9440.

She states that presently PectaSol is the only MCP she has seen that meets the specifications needed for effective results.

Alzheimer's—Autism—Could they have the same roots?

Theories are the seeds of research. Recently an old theory became more plausible as it related to the relationship between mercury, aluminum and other toxic metals as leading to autism, Alzheimer's and Parkinson's disease. Physician and researcher, Dr. Amy Yasko, posited the theory. Yasko is author of a recently published book, "The Puzzle of Autism," has treated autism for years and it would appear she has been able to pinpoint the nexus between several factors and the onset of the condition.

Yasko discovered a genetic factor that results in a defect in the biochemical process known as methylation. Methylation converts folic acid into a food for cell repair and division of cells. According to Dr. Yasko, most people with the genetic defect can detoxify toxins such as heavy metals as long as they don't encounter too many toxins that overload the system. She states that about 20% of the population has this defect, however, only a portion of them develop autism or other neurological disorders.

Dr. Yasko believes the toxins in childhood vaccinations, the mercury (thimerosal) in flu and other adult vaccinations as well as the mercury in fish that we eat regularly, are the keys that help provide the answers. Thimerosal is added to vaccines as a preservative. This is a controversial viewpoint, however, the results she has been attaining with her new method of removing the mercury, as well as the subsequent results of her treatment, solidify her theory that mercury and the genetic inability to properly process folic acid, are major factors in the onset of such brain diseases.

Dr. Robert Jay Rowen writes about Dr. Yasko in his April and May 2005 newsletter, "Second Opinion." Rowen writes in the May issue that Yasko has also developed specific RNA (ribonucleic acid) products to work along with the metal removal. She and Dr. Rowen are both having success in treating autism with both DMPS and her RNA formulas…He also writes about Rashid Buttar, M.D., a physician who treats heavy metal poisoning.

Chelation therapy using EDTA as a chelation agent, removes heavy metals, but does not always elicit desired results; however, there is a newer method that allows a substance known as DMPS (Sodium 2,3-dimercaptopropane-1-sulfonate) to enter the system through the skin to help in assisting in the removal of mercury. DMPS is an agent that targets mercury. Dr. Rowen writes of the experiences of German physician Dr. Dietrich Kinghardt, who has had astonishing results in removing mercury in children with the transdermal (TD) DMPS. It does not have to be taken through an IV and is applied directly to the skin which contains nerves that transport the DMPS into the system.

Dr. Rowen also makes the comment, "And what you may find especially surprising is that the underlying causes of the childhood autism epidemic are the same causes of Alzheimer's disease and Parkinson's disease." These findings of the newer substance DMPS and the linkage to the methylation process that causes some of us to retain heavy metals, may well quickly lead to answers for healing many brain diseases in addition to autism.

Dr. Nan Kathryn Fuchs wrote of a special type of modified citrus pectin (MCP) that was used to help prevent and treat Alzheimer's as well as cancers. The interesting correlation between DMPS and MCP is that both help the body eliminate heavy metals. MCP also creates a condition known as anti-angiogenesis which blocks tumor growth. All of these findings should lend themselves to an even greater understanding that many brain diseases are most likely linked to heavy metal poisoning and not age. Of course, any of these treatments should be conducted under the supervision of an integrated physician.

To learn more about Dr. Amy Yasko and her treatment for autism, go to: www.autismanswer.com.

Alzheimer's—Can triglycerides play a role?

According to Dr. James Balch, a toxic protein called beta amyloid is a major culprit. He says the answer could be simple as he points to high triglycerides as a factor that causes the brain to overload with beta amyloid that he says leads to the formation of plaque in the brain.

Balch points to refined carbohydrates that turn to sugar as a cause for high triglycerides and suggests we avoid simple sugars as much as possible. He also suggests limiting red meat and supplementing with fish oil to prevent Alzheimer's.

He relates a study in which diets of high DHA (docosahexaenoic acid) a fat in fish oil, reduced the deposits of beta amyloid by 70% in mice that were "genetically destined" to have Alzheimer's. Additionally, he pointed to those with higher levels of omega-3 fatty acids as having had better brain function.

A fraction of the sugar cane known as policosanol was proven effective in reducing triglycerides as well. It also raised levels of the good cholesterol known as HDL by as much as 17 percent. Another nutrient he suggests we take to reduce triglycerides is niacin. He recommends "no flush" niacin.

Your physician may already have the above information. If not, you may wish to further research and bring the data to him/her.

ANTIBIOTIC OVER USE: DOES IT CAUSE CANCER?

We are pretty much aware of the downside of antibiotic over use. Antibiotics have been virtual wonder drugs in the past. Today, because of antibiotic overuse for minor disorders and flu symptoms, a new generation of super-bugs has been created. The major concern is that the drugs destroy friendly bacteria as well as healthy cells. Doctors have become aware of the need to replace the friendly bacteria in the intestines with acidophilus and the possibility we may build up an immunity to antibiotics.

The Centers for Disease Control and Prevention have warned physicians to be careful in prescribing antibiotics because of these more recent revelations.

Recently, I spoke with a physician/researcher about the coming new super-bugs. That physician surprised me with the statement that the super-bugs are not "coming," but rather, "they are already here!"

Add to that revelation, the new and more foreboding news about the possible association of antibiotic overuse linked with increased incidence of breast cancer and heart attacks. In the February, 2004 issue of the *Journal of the American Medical Association*, several new studies were cited showing that overuse of antibiotics does more physical harm than initially believed.

An increased incidence of breast cancer is a newer concern for women who have regularly taken antibiotics over the years. In one study of over 10,000 women who had been on antibiotics cumulatively for 500 days over a 17 year period showed twice the risk of breast cancer among antibiotic using women as those women who had not taken any antibiotics. Women, who had not taken quite as much as 500 cumulative days, were also at a higher risk of about 1.5 times more likely to get breast cancer. Additionally, studies will have to be conducted to see if the correlation translates to other cancers as well. This gave me a very uncomfortable feeling since I was one of those young moms who took antibiotics with the mistaken thought in mind that they were a cure-all.

There was no question the study showed more breast cancer risk among women taking the most antibiotics, but the study also cautioned that other factors might be involved when drawing those conclusions. According to the researchers, factors that should be considered are that antibiotics destroy the friendly bacteria in the intestines making proper digestion of foods and the absorption of nutrients more difficult. Another suggestion was that women with existing weakened immune systems end up with more infections, hence, they require more antibiotic therapy. Another consideration is that antibiotics may affect immune response to inflammation and this interference may also be a factor that leads to creating an environment conducive to formation of cancers.

While it was not listed in the study, many alternative physicians have been concerned for years about the ingestion of chlorinated water because chlorine is a gas that also kills bacteria and possibly even good bacteria. In addition, they feel chlorine and other chemicals should not be ingested, especially because many of these chemicals become negatively synergistic when they are combined. The booming sales of water filters are an indication that many Americans already realize the dangers of unfiltered tap water.

The key is to make certain antibiotics are truly indicated for whatever condition arises or work with an integrative physician to use herbs, such as olive leaf extract or a genuine oregano. Even pure fresh garlic has antimicrobial properties.

AORTIC ANEURYSM—WHAT ARE THE SIGNS?

John Ritter's untimely death brought awareness of a condition known as aortic aneurysm. It strikes without warning. The topic of aortic aneurysm was covered in the press, however, very little was written regarding symptoms, early detection and treatment. Many are stricken with aortic aneurysm every year. Unless an autopsy is performed these deaths may summarily be diagnosed and written off as heart attacks.

I would like to attempt to focus on measures that medical professionals have detailed listing steps that are taken to diagnose or treat both thoracic and abdominal aortic aneurysm.

Dr. Stephen Sinatra writes that aortic aneurysm is estimated to be the 13th most common cause of death in the country. He states that there are approximately 5.9 cases per every 100,000 people. The average age of diagnosis is 59 to 69. When aortic aneurysm occurs in young people, it generally occurs due to a genetic factor, says the cardiologist. He states that even seasoned physicians can sometimes miss the diagnosis soon enough to effectively treat the patient. Once the aorta tears, death can occur within up to two hours unless there is an immediate intervention.

In explaining the condition he states, "Individuals with a predisposition to aortic aneurysm develop premature necrosis, or cell death, of the medial (middle) layer of their aorta. In this condition, a loss of elastic fibers and smooth muscle cells leads to the accelerated aging of the aorta, rendering the artery weak and vulnerable to dissection." He also states there is a known association between aortic aneurysms and two fairly rare medical syndromes. They are Marfan's (congenital) and Turner (chromosomal) syndromes. He suggests that people with these diagnosed conditions request their physicians assess them for aortic aneurysm risk. For those with undiagnosed aortic aneurysm, Sinatra states, a serious rise in blood pressure can exacerbate or even cause the tearing of an aneurysm. This fact provides us with all the more cause to mellow out.

Early detection of these silent killers gives a physician the ability to either closely monitor or refer the patient for surgical intervention. Sinatra points to Yale University studies that have indicated the size of the aneurysm would generally determine the form of treatment. He points out, however, regardless of size, once an aneurysm has dissected (torn) immediate surgical intervention is required.

Sinatra lists symptoms of thoracic aortic aneurysm as including constant, nagging or intermittent pain in the neck, chest or upper back; blood in the mucus;

persistent coughing, or a "goose cough" with brassy quality; difficulty swallowing and hoarseness.

Symptoms of abdominal aortic aneurysm include persistent or intermittent pain in the lower abdomen and lower back; a throbbing sensation in the abdomen, which sometimes can be seen or felt as a throbbing lump, which may be accompanied by weight and loss of appetite. The best methods used to detect aneurysm, according to Sinatra, are through ultrasound and trans-esophageal echocardiography, CT scan, MRI or MRA. The simple ultrasound test is available once a year in most areas. The non-invasive screening costs about $99.00 for aortic aneurysm screening, carotid artery screening and extremity blood flow measurements. It takes about 10 minutes. Life Line Screening of Cleveland, Ohio offers it. They set up their ultrasound equipment in local communities. I had the screening two years ago. Life Line Screening can be reached at 216-581-6556.

Among the hospitals Dr. Sinatra feels are best equipped for treating aortic aneurysm, include Cleveland Clinic in Cleveland, Ohio, The Mayo Clinic, Rochester, Mn., Massachusetts General, Boston, Ma, Brigham and Women's Hospital, Boston, Ma, Duke University, Durham, N.C. and Johns Hopkins Hospital in Baltimore, Md.

ARTHRITIS—ARE GLUCOSAMINE & CHONDROITIN INCOMPLETE?

One of the best researchers I am aware of is Dr. David Williams. It was Dr. Williams who first wrote of the benefits of Sambucol for flu symptoms and I've never been without the product since. He was also the one who turned our family onto Xlear Nasal Wash with Xylitol for prevention of colds and flu. Lately he has been writing about the incomplete nature of glucosamine and chondroitin supplements for joint pain and arthritis and has produced a product that he feels provides much more pain relief and joint mobility than glucosamine and chondroitin alone. While Williams supports the use of glucosamine and chondroitin for renewing cartilage, he feels there are a group of other substances that must augment the G & C, to make them work more effectively.

It was especially interesting to me because one of the more general comments I hear about straight glucosamine and chondroitin is that it either doesn't work or takes too long to kick in. Typically, natural methods may take a little longer, but some of those suffering with joint pain, who wisely seek more natural methods of healing, have been disappointed in the overall results of straight glucosamine and chondroitin. I've also heard from those who have found glucosamine and chondroitin to be very effective, which is wonderful news.

Glucosamine and chrondroitin are only part of the quotient, according to Williams. There are many more such compounds found in joint tissue and they should be used along with glucosamine, chondroitin, and other anti-inflammatory herbs, claims Dr. Williams.

Herbal Assistance

Some of the herbs Williams feels are most effective for joint rebuilding, stiffness and joint pain, are grown in Australia. One such herb is Australian Lemon Myrtle, which contains citral, a natural joint cleanser, according to Williams. He points out that normal lemon oil contains three percent citral, while Australian Lemon Myrtle contains 98% citral. Another herb he believes helps joint mobility is Australian Aniseed Mrytle, which has proven effective in easing joint stiffness. Australian Mountain Pepper, he says, eases swelling, and another ingredient, Wild Rosella, is a powerful antioxidant.

Williams feels that additional ingredients such as white willow bark, which contains salicin (aspirin is made from white willow bark); a pain reliever, boswellia extract, feverfew leaf; which stops the body from creating histamines that cause swelling, and devil's claw, which he says, doctors in Europe routinely prescribe for joint discomfort. (According to Williams, feverfew is nature's antihistamine). He states celery seed, another antioxidant, and yucca root, which contains steroidal saponins help alleviate that "stiff" joint feeling. The product he created contains all of the above as well as a little bromelain and papain, both digestive enzymes to help users assimilate the product.

So why would I write about this product? Because I doubt you will ever hear about it in the conventional medical community since it is not a pharmaceutical drug and there are not billions of dollars available to advertise the product.

As I stated early on, David Williams is one of the most informed researchers I have happened upon. His newsletter has always been exceptionally helpful to my own family when looking for natural healing.

Many pharmaceutical, and even over-the-counter, drugs have side-effects and can actually exacerbate other health conditions while relieving pain. My purpose is to present the alternative methods and products in order to allow readers and their physicians to explore the more natural roads to healing. I think it is important to explain that I receive neither financial benefit nor freebies for any product I bring to the attention of readers. My family's own experiences, as well as that of friends and acquaintances, with the negative effects of so many pharmaceutical drugs, has provided the impetus for my seeking out effective, natural means of healing. There may be times when pharmaceuticals are needed, but it is best to reserve those drugs only for those very special occasions. We are living in an age where there is a drug for everything.

For those who are interested in Dr. Williams product, Joint Advantage, you can call 1-800-888-1415. If you would be interested in his monthly newsletter, you can ask about it when you order. A one month supply is about $25.00 and he suggests that you should feel results within one week.

If you are presently taking pharmaceuticals or any other over-the-counter drugs, it's best to first speak with your doctor about trying Joint Advantage.

ASPARTAME: THE STORY ISN'T SWEET

It was a beautiful fall day in the late 1980's. I decided to enjoy biking through the neighborhood, when a friend motioned me over to chat. I was thirsty and she handed me a diet soda. Within minutes after drinking the soda I experienced an anxious "jump out of your skin" feeling.

I never associated the feeling to diet drinks until the exact reaction occurred several weeks later when I drank yet, another can of diet soda. Once the unusual anxiety returned, I immediately asked what was in the soda. "Aspartame," she stated. I chalked it up to a severe allergy or hypersensitivity to aspartame and avoided the substance and went about my life. However, several years later, the same reaction occurred when I inadvertently drank a lemonade drink containing aspartame. It made me curious as to what could cause such a reaction.

Over the years since my experiences, I have studied both the pros and cons of aspartame.

The basic argument supporting its safety is that it was approved by the Food & Drug Administration (FDA) after numerous studies showed it to be safe. Another argument is that these components are all natural occurring substances in both plant and human life.

In order to maintain perspective, one must keep in mind the batting average of the FDA when it comes to the approval of medications. The authors of "Worst Pills/Best Pills," state, "there are 100,000 deaths a year from adverse drug reactions; each year approximately 1.5 million people in the United States are injured so seriously by adverse drug reactions, that they require hospitalization." These deaths and adverse reactions are all caused by drugs officially approved by the

FDA. All of these drugs were also tested to be safe and subsequently approved—then many were withdrawn from the market.

What is Aspartame?

Aspartame contains 50 percent phenylalanine, 40 percent aspartic acid and 10 percent methanol. Neurosurgeon, Dr. Russell Blaylock, writes, in his book, *Excitotoxins: The Taste That Kills*, that the manner in which the excitatory amino acids and methanol in aspartame, break down, they are toxic to the central nervous system and can exacerbate neurological disorders and, over time, even create symptoms of neurological disorders. He describes aspartame as a neurotoxin. Additionally, he states that one in 50 people either have, or carry the gene for phenylketonuria (PKU), a genetic disease wherein phenylalanine cannot be metabolized. Those people, he says, are adversely affected by the phenylalanine in aspartame. Dr. Blaylock further states that the methanol in diet drinks essentially converts to "wood alcohol," formaldehyde and formic acid where it can also affect the optic nerve.

Questioning the safety studies

Ohio psychiatrist, Ralph G. Walton, M.D., Chairman and professor of Psychiatry at Northeastern Ohio Universities, College of Medicine, was prompted to review and analyze the aspartame studies. He took his investigation a step further and traced the source of funding for each of the studies. His examination revealed that of 164 studies on aspartame, there were 90 independent studies not sponsored by industry sources. He found that 92 percent of these studies, identified one or more problems with aspartame. Not surprisingly, when he examined the 74 studies sponsored by the industry-related sources, he noted that 100 percent of those studies found no problem with aspartame. This troubled the doctor.

Dr. Walton's observations

I contacted Dr. Walton, in an effort to learn what prompted his interest in the effects of aspartame. He explained that his first indication of a problem with aspartame occurred, when one of his patients suffered a grand mal seizure with no apparent cause. After conducting intensive medical tests, there was still no answer for her seizure. After the seizure, the patient also experienced mania, insomnia and irritability. In examining her daily habits closely, Dr. Walton discovered that the only substantial change in her habits had been a switch from sugar to aspartame several weeks prior to her grand mal seizure. The curious doctor then attempted to collect further information on other such medical anomalies. The common thread he discovered was the heavy use of aspartame among patients suffering unexplained grand mal seizures, depression and anxiety. Also, of interest was that shortly after his patient with the grand mal seizure discontinued all aspartame use, she suffered no further episodes of seizures, mania or insomnia.

Dr. Walton then conducted his own double-blind studies among people with a tendency toward anxiety. His studies found that both anxiety and depression were greatly exacerbated among those in the aspartame ingesting group. Additionally, another unfortunate finding of his study was that two people in the aspartame group, suffered intra-ocular bleeding. He attributes this to the 10 percent methanol in aspartame. He now advises all of his patients to avoid any products containing aspartame. Dr.Walton also expressed additional concern about brain chemistry changes as well as interactions between various medications and aspartame.

Neurosurgeon, Russell Blaylock, M.D. sees aspartame as causing serious cumulative neurological side-effects for all users. Blaylock explains that many who use aspartame products show no immediate side-effects. He states that quite frequently, neurological problems surface only after a period of use, although people with existing neurological disorders or hypersensitivities will display more immediate symptoms. He frets that most doctors fail to consider an association between aspartame and neurological disorders due to lack of information available within the conventional medical community.

When I asked Dr. Blaylock what he would like to convey to readers regarding the use of aspartame, his most urgent admonition was that pregnant women avoid using products containing aspartame, because aspartame concentrates in the placenta causing excessive exposure to the unborn child. He feels young children using aspartame are at higher risk for neurological and other physical symptoms because they will have been exposed to it for many more years than today's adults who only began using it in the 1980's. It may be years before the dangers of aspartame are realized, claims Dr. Blaylock.

H. J. Roberts, M.D. expresses concern

Diabetes specialist, H. J. Roberts, endocrinologist and member of the Endocrine Society, the American Federation for Clinical Research and The American College of Physicians, agrees with Walton and Blaylock and those researchers who express concerns about neurological damage as well as problems with glucose control and optic nerve damage. Roberts has authored several books on aspartame. "Aspartame Disease: An Ignored Epidemic," is among those publications. Roberts asserts that aspartame when mixed with certain classes of drugs, can enhance those drugs while diminishing the effects of others. We have recently learned that something as simple as grapefruit juice, when taken with certain medications, can create serious reactions, so it is not unthinkable that the same could be the case with any substance, including aspartame. In an interview, Dr. Roberts stated, "Clinically, we have seen interactions with a group of drugs such as Propanolol, Coumadin, and others, when combined with aspartame."

I visited many industry-related web sites and their arguments sounded convincing—it's natural—studies show it is safe—and the FDA approved it. Convincing—unless one were to examine the background of its approval, which is outlined in her compelling book, "Deadly Deception," by medical researcher, Mary Nash Stoddard. She reconstructs the road to approval and outlines problems associated with the approval of aspartame. She explains that a Public Board of Inquiry voted to ban aspartame because of studies indicating mutagenic (cancer causing) effects and brain tumors in aspartame-fed mice, yet, the chairman of the FDA, nonetheless, ordered its approval for beverages in 1983. Within months of approval, that FDA official took a position with the public relations firm representing the pharmaceutical company manufacturing aspartame, according to Stoddard. She relates how negative research findings were disclosed to the FDA only after approval had been granted. She states many of the test animals developed large tumors but were not reported to the FDA. The book is a must-read for all users of aspartame.

The game of musical chairs between FDA and pharmaceutical industry employees is nothing new. These conflicts of interest, along with perks to some physicians, will continue to make it difficult to acquire totally objective studies on many new drugs as well as food additives such as aspartame. What makes aspartame of special concern is that a prescription is not necessary. You may ingest it without even realizing it in any number of foods and drinks.

For further information you can check out various web sites. I found one especially helpful in giving a point-by-point response to aspartame industry claims:

Mark Gold at holisticmed.com/aspartame. Other excellent sites are mercola.com, key word "aspartame;" dorway.com which has posted reports and provides many other related links. Rich Murray, rmforall@att.net lists sites as well as "cites."

I'm not Carrie Nation and I have no desire to snatch aspartame products off grocery shelves if consumers wish to use them. I merely feel that health-conscious readers have a right to information on both sides of this issue. The fact is, there are a great many highly respected medical professionals and researchers opposed to aspartame use, quite contrary to what the urban legend sites and aspartame-related special interests are claiming. Find out for yourself.

BLADDER INFECTIONS? STUDY SAYS CIPRO IS NOT THE ANSWER

A study involving the treatment of 13,000 women suffering the discomfort of acute urinary tract infections (bladder infections) was cited in the June issue of Worst Pills/Best Pills newsletter. The study concluded that most women do not receive the proper treatment for bladder infections. Astonishingly, only 37 percent of the women in the study had been prescribed the first-choice drugs for the condition. The preferred treatment is the combination antibiotic (trimethoprim/sulfamethoxazole) Bactrim, Septra or Cotrim It is considered a sulfa drug so those who cannot tolerate sulfa drugs would necessarily be prescribed an appropriate alternative.

Another 32 percent in the same study were prescribed the fluoroquinolone antibiotic (ciprofloxacin) Cipro, a drug, according to the authors, is not considered the first-choice treatment for such infections. Cipro, if you will remember, is effective against anthrax. It is a very strong antibiotic for use among individuals with infections resistant to other antibiotics. It has the potential of serious side effects such as creating tendonitis, Achilles' tendonitis including tendon rupture as well as central nervous system problems including psychosis. A rare side effect is collapse of the circulatory system. Patients using Aminophylline or theophylline medications must have their doses adjusted when taking Cipro. Another finding of the study was that the recommended duration of treatment for acute bladder infections is just three days, yet the most common duration among the women was 10 days followed by seven and then five.

Researchers for the Federal Centers for Disease Control are concerned that the overuse of antibiotics has been resulting in a nation overflowing with antibiotic resistance. Resistance means the pills won't work when you really need them.

Additionally, the overuse of antibiotics creates an overgrowth of yeast that sets you up for a yeast infection. Additionally, Cipro can be five to seven times more costly than other equally effective antibiotics.

The question is: What can I do if I have a bladder infection—or any infection? If you choose the conventional route, you can help reduce your chances of becoming drug resistant by insisting your physician conduct a culture and sensitivity (C&S) test. The bacteria specimen is sent to a laboratory where the bacteria present are isolated and grown for 48 hours. The lab then tests to see exactly which antibiotics kill the bacteria. They can also tell which antibiotics don't work against your specific bacteria. Many times, inexpensive antibiotics are capable of fighting the infection. A C&S assures you are not exposed to needless antibiotics. Whether using conventional treatment or alternative, you should always supplement your antibiotic with a probiotic. The body's "friendly bacteria", essential for digestion and other body functions, should always be replaced because antibiotics kill both bad and our "friendly bacteria."

Drinking lots of pure water provides tremendous assistance to the bladder by helping to flush bacteria out. Both conventional and alternative physicians suggest cranberry juice. It should be obtained from a health food store. Yesterday, I spent time reading the labels of every "cranberry juice" product on the grocery store shelf and most had fillers and were loaded with sugar and corn syrup, apple and grape juice. All had very little cranberry content. Cranberry juice at the health food store is bitter because it is pure and concentrated. It should be diluted with pure water as instructed. You may not like the taste, but it works well to flush the system to create an environment that inhibits the adherence and proliferation of bacteria in the bladder. The substance that makes cranberry juice so effective is d-mannose, a natural occurring sugar that inhibits bacteria from reproducing in the bladder. D-mannose creates a "slippery" wall that washes bacteria from the bladder. For those with gout or those who cannot otherwise take cranberry juice, d-mannose can be purchased from the health food store.

Antibiotic resistance is a scary thing and it is of great concern to national health officials. It will be up to you to protect your family from consuming unnecessary drugs. When it comes to pharmaceutical interests, learn to delineate for yourself the fine line between necessity and market share.

Please read the article listed below for the latest findings on Cipro

Latest findings on Cipro

Would you believe a class of antibiotics could cause Achilles' tendon ruptures? Would you believe that same class of antibiotics could cause peripheral neuropathies? Peripheral neuropathies can involve muscle weakness, paresthesias, impaired reflexes and autonomic symptoms in the hands and feet. Neuropathy generally occurs in patients with diabetes mellitus, kidney disease or liver disease. A neuropathy is considered any disease of the nerves or injury to nerves. It can also occur in patients taking any of the fluoroquinolone class of drugs and other drugs.

Alternative physicians have been highly suspicious of these seemingly unassociated conditions for quite some time, however, the association between Fluoroquinolone antibiotics such as (Cipro, Tequin, Avelox, Factive, Floxin, Levaquin, Maxaquin, Noroxin, Penetrex, Trovan and Zagam), has now been confirmed. There will be a warning on all of the above antibiotics in the future. Achilles' tendon ruptures as well as rotator cuff tendon; biceps and hand tendons have also been involved according to the authors of *Worst Pills/Best Pills.*

These warnings are important since most all of us are subject to commercials touting the great benefits of numerous new drugs that have subsequently been yanked from the market.

BLADDER INFECTION: WHAT IS THE NATURAL ANSWER?

Dr. Jonathon Wright is one of the most well-known alternative doctors in the United States. He has authored *"Dr. Wright's Book of Nutritional Therapy,"* as well as books on prostate health, menopause and he has established a guide to locating nutrition minded physicians. Dr. Wright has been at the forefront of the movement to petition the Federal Drug Administration to place warnings on statin drugs explaining that statin drugs such as Lipitor, Zocor and Pravachol, etc., deplete coenzyme Ql0 an enzyme essential to heart health. He also writes for "Prevention Magazine."

Natural bladder infection treatment

He has also written papers on his use of a common substance to treat bladder infections and urinary tract infections. His recommendations may be helpful to millions of Americans who have had bouts with common urinary tract infections (UTI's). What makes his treatment so illuminating is that his cure for bladder infections is not an antibiotic and is actually a substance that is beneficial to the body. It is known as D-Mannose; a form of simple sugar closely related to glucose, but that metabolizes differently than glucose. The manner in which it metabolizes is exactly what makes it so effective in fighting urinary tract infections.

D-Mannose is a naturally occurring simple sugar. Our bodies metabolize only a small amount of the D-Mannose, and the larger balance is excreted through the urine. How does this help fight bladder and urinary tract infections? The type of bladder infections most women suffer, is caused by an e-coli germ that finds its way into the urinary tract. The D-Mannose interacts because its chemical structure binds itself to the type of e-coli bacteria found in over 90% of all bladder infections, according to Dr. Wright. Since the larger portion of the D-Mannose binds itself to the bacteria, making the bacteria ineffective, it then washes out of the system during urination. Dr. Wright explains that D-Mannose has been extremely effective for his patients because it works all the way back to the kidneys, traveling through the system, where it binds the unwanted bacteria and washes it out of the body through drinking and elimination. For those patients with chronic urinary tract infections, he prescribes small amounts on a daily basis as "preventive maintenance."

Dr. Wright states that by using D-Mannose, especially with women and young girls, it additionally avoids the formation of yeast infections generally caused by antibiotic therapy. Antibiotics allow yeast to proliferate because they kill off the "friendly" bacteria that is so essential to normal body function. Dr. Wright states that "Long term or often repeated antibiotic use can lead to major disruptions in normal body microflora, and sometimes to major disruptions in health, especially immune system function. (It is suspected that "killer" E.coli of recent years are "mutants" caused by persistent antibiotic feeding to animals)."

Cranberry Juice

D-Mannose can be found in cranberry juice, however, commercial cranberry juices have such high concentrations of fructose and other sugars, they may not be as helpful. Cranberry juice alone does not act as efficiently as D-Mannose when taken alone, but it does help, according to Wright. A natural unsweetened cranberry juice can be found at the health food store in more concentrated form but be prepared—even when you dilute it—it's bitter tasting!

For those who wish to avoid the bitterness of cranberry, I have located several sources for D-Mannose for those readers who may be interested in seeking more information about it or would like to order it. Progressive Laboratories is one source at 800-527-9512, and Tahoma Clinic (Dr. Wright is associated with the clinic) at 425-264-0051, also listed was WebWide Marketing in Folsom, California—Toll-Free 888-779-7177.

BLOOD TESTS: WHY DO WE NEED THEM?

The doctor hands you a sheet with check marks on it. You take the sheet to the laboratory and they draw your blood. You then wait for the doctor to tell you the results of your tests. They generally tell you the test results were okay or you should take more medications and change your diet based on the results of those tests. You should know what those tests mean. It's a good idea to request copies to keep in your own home health files. You can compare test results yourself, and even more important, should you change physicians, you can pass along the results of your past regular blood work. It can be helpful to your new doctor and can be a source for determining trends as each blood value goes up or down. I used my Taber's Medical dictionary as well as the web site of Joseph Mercola, D.O. and the medical encyclopedia online to obtain information on the meaning of blood tests.

So what does your blood test show?

Glucose: (sugar) is important in helping you maintain energy. Values of over 105 after fasting 12 hours can suggest you are on the road to diabetes. Higher levels over 120 during non-fasting blood draws can be an indicator of future diabetes.

Sodium: (electrolyte—electric conducting) Salt and water balance is important. Low levels can indicate too much water intake, heart failure and kidney failure. High levels can indicate not enough water is being taken or salt intake is too high.

Potassium: (electrolyte—electric conducting) Low levels may mean severe diarrhea, alcoholism or diuretics (water pills) are being taken without replenishing with potassium supplements. Low levels can lead to muscle and heart weakness.

Magnesium: Probably one of the most important, yet overlooked, minerals. Magnesium triggers the function of over 350 enzymes in the body and is essential to healthy heart function. Low levels can lead to heart irregularities, constipation, and nervous disorders such as anxiety.

Calcium: Calcium is involved in bone metabolism, protein absorption, fat transfer, muscle contraction, and transmission of nerve impulses, blood clotting, and heart function.

Chloride: An electrolyte (electric conducting) controlled by the kidneys that help our bodies maintain an acid-based balance. It assists in the regulation of blood volume and artery pressure. High levels can indicate acidosis.

BUN (Blood Urea Nitrogen): BUN is a waste product from protein breakdown in the liver. Kidney damage, too much protein, inadequate fluid intake, various drugs, intestinal bleeding, exercise, heart failure or inadequate digestive enzyme output by the pancreas, can cause increases. Decreased levels are most commonly due to inadequate protein intake, malabsorption, or liver damage.

Creatinine: Creatinine is another protein breakdown product. It relates to muscle mass. Low levels are commonly seen in inadequate protein intake, liver disease, kidney damage or pregnancy. High levels may indicate kidney damage.

Uric Acid: Indicates purine metabolism. High levels are seen in gout, infections, high protein diets, and kidney disease. Low levels generally indicate protein and molybdenum (trace mineral) deficiency, liver damage or an overly acidic kidney.

Phosphate: Phosphate is important in bone development. Most of the phosphate in the body is found in the bones. Phosphate levels are essential to muscle and nerve operation. Low levels in the blood can be associated with starvation or malnutrition. Low levels can lead to muscle weakness. High levels in the blood can usually associated with kidney disease.

Albumen: This protein is made in the liver. It binds toxic waste products, and dangerous drugs that might damage the body. It also helps control the exact amount of water in our tissues. It serves to transport vitamins, minerals and hormones. The higher this number is, the better. The highest one can reasonably expect would be 5.5.

Alkaline Phosphatase: Alkaline phosphatase is an enzyme present in all body tissue. It is found in bone, liver, bile ducts and the gut. High levels in the blood may indicate bone, liver or bile duct disease. Certain drugs may also cause high levels. Low levels indicate low functioning adrenal glands, protein deficiency, malnutrition or more commonly, a deficiency in zinc.

Gamma-Glutamyl tranferase (GGT): Amino acid found in the liver. Will rise with alcohol use, liver disease, or excess magnesium. Decreased levels can be found in hypothyroidism and more commonly decreased magnesium levels.

Transaminases (SGTP) & (SGOT): Enzymes primarily found in the liver. Increases with excessive alcohol, certain drugs, liver disease and bile duct disease. Hepatitis can raise these levels. According to Dr. Mercola, "Low levels of GGTP may indicate a magnesium deficiency. Low levels of SGPT and SGOT may indicate deficiency of vitamin B6."

Lactate Dehydrogenase (LDH): LDH is an enzyme found in all tissues in the body. Again, Dr. Mercola states, "A high level in the blood can result from a number of different diseases. Also, slightly elevated levels in the blood are common and usually do not indicate disease. The most common sources of LDH are the heart, liver, muscles, and red blood cells."

Total Protein: A measure of the total amount of protein in your blood. High or low protein counts generally indicate that a physician should conduct more intricate testing for specific diseases.

Iron: Iron is necessary to make hemoglobin and to help transfer oxygen to the muscle. Iron too low or iron too high may both result in fatigue. Mercola suggests that low iron results should be followed by Ferritin test, especially menstruating females.

Triglycerides: These are fats used as fuel by the body, and as an energy source for metabolism. According to Mercola again, "Increased levels are almost always a sign of too much carbohydrate intake. Decreased levels are seen in hyperthyroidism, malnutrition and malabsorption."

Cholesterol: Group of fats vital to cell membranes, nerve fibers and bile salts, and a necessary precursor for the sex hormones.

LDL (cholesterol): LDL is the "bad cholesterol" that, in excess amounts, attaches to artery walls and tissue.

HDL (cholesterol) HDL is the "good cholesterol" that prevents narrowing of the artery walls by removing the excess cholesterol and excreting it through the liver. The higher the better.

CO2: CO_2 levels are related to the respiratory exchange of carbon dioxide in the lungs.

WBC: White blood count measures the total number of white blood cells. Your white blood cells kill bacteria. High levels generally indicate infection. Other more serious diseases can be spotted through a high WBC or low count.

Hemoglobin: Hemoglobin is important to provide the transport of oxygen and carbon in the blood. It is used to detect anemia, poor diet or malabsorption.

Hematocrit: Measures percentage of red blood cells in whole blood. Overhydration or anemia show reduced levels. Dehydration shows elevated levels. **MCV:** Measurement of average size of the red blood cells and their volume in the blood. Used to measure for iron deficiency, rheumatoid arthritis, or B12 or folic acid deficiency.

BREAST CANCER—ALTERNATIVE VIEWS ON CAUSES AND CURES ALUMINUM CONNECTION?

A recent nightly news segment focused on a study indicating there may be a possible link between breast cancer and the use of anti-perspirants. The retrospective study conducted by Chicago physician Kris McGrath, M.D., was of special interest to me because the issue of aluminum in anti-perspirants has created a contentious debate for over 30 years. It made sense to me and I began using non-aluminum containing deodorants more than 20 years ago. There was a major concern among integrative and alternative physicians about suppressing sweating, a normal body function, through the use of aluminum chlorhydrate.

I contacted Dr. McGrath to learn more about his study. He too, feels a major offending culprit appears to be aluminum chlorhydrate, the ingredient that suppresses perspiration. McGrath, admits there are other environmental causes of breast cancer, however, he is convinced that because at least 50 percent of breast cancer cases have no known cause, he is on the right track by considering the possibility that aluminum salts in anti-perspirants may be a possible factor.

McGrath's small study included many underlying components. Mainly, he was curious about why most breast tumors occurred in the upper outer quadrant of the breast—the area of the axilla (arm-pit) where women apply anti-perspirants. He was also concerned that the absorption of aluminum was greater among women who applied anti-perspirants immediately after shaving their armpits. Shaving disrupts the dermal layer, allowing easier exposure to and absorption of the aluminum, according to McGrath. He suggests that intensity and length of usage may also be a factor to consider in determining overall exposure.

McGrath's study also notes the importance of pH changes in the skin area of the axilla, which take place with daily use of anti-perspirants. Small changes in pH can affect the concentrations of aluminum on the skin. The pH alterations create an acidic environment in the under arm area similar to "acid rain," according to McGrath. McGrath believes this may partially explain why under-developed nations who practice different hygiene habits (no anti-perspirant use, I assume,) experience fewer cases of breast cancer. His report also brings into focus the significance between the lymphatic flow that extends from the breast tissue into the underarm area where tumors are formed. Consider that aluminum is contained in many products we consume and has always been felt to be innocuous until recently. It is in antacids, food and many topical skin applications. Perhaps the increase in our usage is overloading our systems. A recent report by the

National Institutes of Environmental Health Sciences acknowledged that flouride was shown to enhance the toxicity of aluminum. Additionally, Kerri Bodmer and Nan Kathyrn Fuchs, PhD, report in "The Giant Book of Women's Health Secrets," that while calcium citrate is a good form of calcium for women, it too, enhances the body's absorption of aluminum.

Our bodies are wonderfully made. They have the ability to eliminate toxins, however, when toxin content overwhelms the system it may place a burden on our immune function.

Aluminum is also being questioned in Alzheimer's disease, since abnormal accumulations of aluminum have been found in Alzheimer's affected brains. Observations have also shown aluminum affects the member performance of animals.

These smaller studies can be easily dismissed, but the fact is, there are no decent comprehensive studies to discount this possibility; and we still have no clue about what causes 50 percent of breast cancer cases. McGrath's report suggests, "Case-control investigation," are now necessary to further evaluate such an association. As with tobacco and lung cancer studies, the intensity of exposure is paramount."

There are many variables and every person's immune system may possess stronger or weaker hypersensitivities to various environmental factors. In the past the main offending culprit appears to be aluminum chlorhydrate, the very ingredient that suppresses perspiration. A recent Report by the National Institutes of Environmental Heath Sciences (NIEHS) acknowledged that fluoride was shown to have synergistic effects on the toxicity of aluminum.

I truly hope Dr. McGrath continues to push for further studies. He has done a great service to those who take his findings into consideration.

I can remember when every victim of Alzheimer's disease I personally knew of, was female. I can also remember a time when only females used anti-perspirants. Perspiring was a manly, sexy thing. Today, many men's deodorants now contain aluminum chlorhydrate as an anti-perspirant agent as well and it's interesting that Alzheimer's is becoming common among men. Since men naturally tend to sweat more than women, the overall effects of the aluminum and pH changes on males may be of even more concern. But then, who's keeping score—that's the problem.

BREAST CANCER—FRACTION OF GINSENG FIGHTS CANCERS

In spite of how well we take care of ourselves, we can contract various diseases. There are some extraneous conditions over which we have no control. The air we breath, the chemicals in the water we drink, the chemicals we use for house cleaning, chemicals in our food, environmental factors, low level radiation and genetics, can all take a toll on our health in one way or another. In fact, some polio shots we received in the 50's and 60's may be carrying a monkey virus that can cause cancer. It was not discovered until the late 1970's and certain batches in certain states, carried the virus. Those things happen. The only thing we can do about it is hope that our immune systems reject these assaults to our systems. We must work to maintain a stronger immune system. For those who already have cancers, there is new information that may help them in their treatment.

Ginseng: The good and the bad

It is widely known that whole ginseng is something a cancer patient should never take. Ginseng can be good for healthy people, because a glucose-formed compound in ginseng, "ginsenosides" causes cell growth and reproduction. Unfortunately, whole ginseng does not differentiate between healthy cells and unhealthy cells in cancer patients and it causes all cells to grow.

New cancer-fighting component isolated in ginseng.

According to Nan Kathryn Fuchs, PhD, editor of "Women's Health," another discovery has been made pertaining to the components of ginseng, and other plant extracts, that when isolated from the cell growth components, can fight cancer cells. The isolated non-glucose-formed compounds in ginseng and other plants known as "aglycon sapogenins" actually have anti-cancer properties. These properties must be separated and isolated from the ginseng in a laboratory. It takes 100 pounds of ginseng to make about one gram of aglycon sapogenins.

Aglycon sapogenins work with and without chemotherapy

Chemotherapy is used to kill cancer cells and it does kill the weakest of cancer cells along with many normal cells. Stronger cancer cells can survive and grow. Cancer cells can become resistant to chemotherapy drugs just as bacteria can become resistant to antibiotics.

According to Dr. Fuchs, a study on ovarian cancer cells showed that when Rh2 (aglycon Sapogenins) was used along with cisplatin, a conventional chemotherapy treatment, "tumors were significantly inhibited and survival increased dramatically. So with or without chemotherapy, these cancer-fighting substances appear to keep working.," states Fuchs.

Japanese study: aglycon sapogenins reversed cancer

A Japanese study conducted in April 1989, using aglycon sapogenins, found that not only did the formula stop liver cancer cells from growing; they actually transformed them back into normal cells. According to Fuchs, the researchers referred to this phenomenon as "reverse transformation" or "decarcinogenesis."

Dr. Fuchs has pointed out that since the discovery of this promising compound, many companies are rushing to sell less expensive weaker forms of the product. That happens frequently when any herb or substance is found to be helpful. Fuchs further explains that the best source for aglycon sapogenins is the Canadian company that supplied the oral formula used in a clinical trial known as the "Harbor-UCLA" trial. The formula used in the trial was called Carseng Oral Solution, a liquid that is more easily absorbed. It is made from standardized ginseng, which is important. The company manufacturing the treatment has worked with plant extracts for many years. That company is Pegasus Pharmaceuticals, a research-based biotech company that specializes in developing pharmaceuticals from plants (604-303-9952). Fuchs claims this particular pharmacuetical has the science behind their research. There is a U.S. distributor for Pegasus Pharmaceuticals in northern California—EcoNugenics, Inc.—a company directed by Dr. Isaac Eliaz, a medical doctor and acupuncturist who specializes in cancer treatment (800-308-5518).

Dr. Fuchs explained "An abstract on the effects of the oral solution has been submitted to ASCO (The American Society of Clinical Oncology) a prestigious medical association." She says she is anxiously awaiting its acceptance and she will inform us of the results once they are shared with oncologists across the U.S.

For those who have their cancers under control, Fuchs says a reduced potency product will soon be available for those who already have their cancers under control. Of course, it will be less expensive than the oral solution. The new product, Carseng-C is expected to become available in a few months. This reduced potency product will be made available in the U.S. through Health Secrets USA (313-56-6800).

Sometimes, a good thing can move slowly. These studies began in 1989 and have finally reached a point where they most probably will be recommended for use as an adjunct to chemotherapy. They can also be used separately. Your doctor may wish to speak with physicians who have used the product or with representatives of the Canadian pharmaceutical.

BROMELAIN—HEALING WITH PINEAPPLE

Believe it or not, we aren't born with "pharmaceutical deficiencies." Sometimes eating something as simple as raw pineapple, or taking bromelain (derived from the pineapple fruit and stem), can do wonders to assist in numerous healing functions.

The inflammation factor, again:

Research is proving that the disease process itself follows a pattern that begins with chronic inflammation. It is currently being acknowledged that even heart disease begins with the inflammation process. There are many amino acids, enzymes and foods that help us avoid inflammation; bromelain is one.

A pioneer of enzyme research, Dr. Edward Howell, points out in a 1986 publication, "*Enzyme Nutrition: The Food Enzyme Concept*," that enzymes are involved in every metabolic process that takes place within our bodies.

According to Howell, enzymes fall into two categories: metabolic and digestive. Dr. Howell posits that we lose enzymes as we age and through highly cooked and processed foods. According to Dr. Howell, when we are deficient in digestive enzymes, we must use our metabolic enzymes to process food, which depletes them for other necessary functions within our body. He states that this deficiency causes our bodies to age more quickly. We need metabolic enzymes to remove fat from our blood vessels, to make hormones, and even to assist us in the thinking process, according to Dr. Howell. His theories and studies point to the importance of eating raw fruits and vegetables.

Bromelain helps prevent platelet aggregation (blood clotting):

One of the many benefits of bromelain is that while it does not necessarily act as a strong blood thinner, it does help to prevent the inflammation process, which leads to platelet aggregation (blood clots). Bromelain smoothes the blood, according to Howell.

Dr. Andrew Weil, a well-known alternative physician, states bromelain is very helpful in treating bruises, sprains and strains by reducing swelling, which alleviates tenderness and pain. Weil says this powerful anti-inflammatory effect of bromelain can also help reduce postoperative swelling. Additionally, the bromelain contained in fresh pineapple can relieve indigestion. Bromelain, according to Weil, helps break down the amino acid bonds in proteins, which promotes good digestion.

Benefits from bromelain:

- Reduces pain, bruising, and swelling from trauma of sports injuries and surgery. It speeds the healing process

- Relieves the symptoms of gastrointestinal upset, aids in the healing of gastric ulcers, and is used as a digestive enzyme for pancreatic insufficiency

- Inhibits blood clot formation and breaks down build-up of plaque in arteries, it is useful for thrombosis, thrombophlebitis, varicose veins, and atherosclerosis.

- Reduces joint inflammation in rheumatoid arthritis, osteoarthritis, sciatica, bursitis, tendinitis, and scleroderma

- Increases the actions of chemotherapy drugs and antibiotics

- Suppresses cough and decreases bronchial secretions, resulting in increased lung function in patients with upper respiratory tract infections. It is also effective in patients with sinusitis.

- Several studies suggest use as an anti-metastatic agent with chemotherapy.

Bromelain is only one of the many enzymes our bodies need and raw foods provide the best sources of our enzymes. An excellent feature of raw pineapple is that it doesn't taste like medicine; it's delicious as well as healing. As always, discuss these matters with your physician.

BURIED EMOTIONS CAN AFFECT YOUR HEALTH

I woke up far too early this morning, and hit the remote to see what was cooking on TV. I was greeted by an infomercial featuring Tony Robbins and his famous smile. He preaches about success and happiness. There he stood, all 32 of his artificially whitened teeth, gleaming in the sun. I like Tony Robbins and think he truly is the picture of success. It just can't get better than making money doing the things you love. He's a true "cheer monger" and that can be good. I love cheerful people. It's just that there are days when I wonder who could possibly be that happy all of the time. The answer: No one. Those "cheer mongers" sometimes make us think something is wrong with us if we aren't always feeling on top of the world. It's an unrealistic expectation.

In the volumes of books and references I found on the benefits of cheer, there was far less reference, conversely, explaining the benefits of having that "good cry." There is no decisive science to explaining the benefits of crying, but it's apparent that certain types of crying are beneficial to many. I'm not speaking of crying from severe depression or unbearable grief, but of an occasional letting of tears when we find ourselves overwhelmed, disappointed, feeling helpless and sad or feeling sorry over the misfortune of others.

An interesting observation I found was that the composition of tears released from slicing an onion is different than that of tears from a truly emotional cry. That has led some researchers to believe that the proteins released in emotional tears may somehow indicate crying can eliminate toxic substances. This could also explain why so many people express relief and explain they feel refreshed after having that good cry.

The issues of human touch and crying have been of interest to me since an experience I once had while working in a medical office. A distraught woman, whose blood pressure had initially been soaring, experienced a tremendous decrease in blood pressure after I hugged her and allowed her to "cry on my shoulder." I often wondered if her sense of calm came from the empathy or the tears, or both.

There are many other references even going back to Aristotle who explained that a good cry was a "cleansing" process. There is something cathartic to the process of crying. It can release tension and clear the cobwebs when things in life become overwhelming.

Now, I'm not speaking of sniveling or hanging out at the Wailing Wall. No one likes sniveling, whining or constant boo-hooing. Sometimes that behavior is a sign of a more serious problem and responds better to professional counselling.

I'm speaking of crying as a form of release and healing.

Somewhere along the line, we Americans adopted a "boys don't cry" attitude that sadly seems to have survived despite the proof of its destructive nature to men and boys. Even the Bible says, "Jesus wept."

One of my favorite actors, Andy Garcia, won my heart and soul for life, the day he appeared before the world, tears streaming down his face, as he plead with then Attorney General, Janet Reno to allow the five-year-old Cuban child, Elian Gonzalez to remain in the United States. I wept right along with Garcia and my respect and admiration for him grew even greater that day. He was not crying for himself, though, he was crying over the plight of the child.

Just like the old song from R.E.M. "Everybody Hurts, Sometime," we need to acknowledge that is a fact for both sexes.

The Holiday season is a time when sadness multiplies for some. Many times, our emotions and problems become magnified during the Holidays. Sometimes we need to shed a few tears before we can get back on track. It sounds like an old bromide, but even after that tearful session, we must reflect on what's good and positive in our lives. It will help us gain a better perspective and help us to grow.

NOTE: It's important to realize that constant feelings of despair are an indicator it's time to seek professional help. In the meantime, there is a neat and simply written book that may help shed light on many issues. It is titled: "<u>Feelings Buried Alive Never Die...</u>" by Karol K. Truman.

During those occasional down times, go ahead and release tears of healing.

CALCIUM CRAZE—MAGNESIUM IS ELEMENTAL FOR BONES

The country is in a calcium craze. Women are constantly being warned of the need for additional calcium and are consuming it in all forms, especially calcium carbonate (chalk). It's the cheapest and most difficult to assimilate. Yet, according to Nan Fuchs, Ph.D., and health researcher, Kerri Bodmer, cases of osteoporosis are increasing. In fact, so are the numbers of women with heart disease, PMS and arthritis. Bodmer and Fuchs are not alone in their belief that taking calcium alone can do more harm than good. They write that calcium without magnesium and vitamin D, may be supplanting itself into our soft tissue. They go so far as to ask the question, "Is calcium the culprit behind the increasing rates of osteoporosis, premenstrual syndrome, arthritis, and heart disease among women?" Sounds strange, doesn't it? Especially since we have been inundated with admonitions to increase calcium intake via supplementation. But then, think about it—haven't these same "experts" been advising us for over 30 years, that we need hormone replacement therapy (HRT) to build strong bone and protect our hearts?

Alternative physicians are concerned that excessive calcium may be improperly absorbed and may interfere with the balance of our magnesium that is extremely essential to heart function.

In their book, *The Giant Book of Women's Health Secrets*, Bodmer and Fuchs state, "Taking more calcium without adequate magnesium—and what is adequate for one woman may be insufficient for another—may either create calcium malabsorption or create a magnesium deficiency." They point to a study reported in "International Clinical Nutrition Review", in which volunteers on a low magnesium diet were given both calcium and vitamin D supplements. All subjects were magnesium-deficient, and all but one became deficient in calcium, as well, in spite of the fact that calcium had also been added to their diet. However, when the women were given magnesium, both their magnesium and calcium blood levels rapidly increased. Another published study in the *Journal of Applied Nutrition* showed women who increased magnesium and took less calcium, actually showed an increase in bone density. Additionally, Bodmer and Fuchs posit that magnesium helps to regulate the increase in calcitonin and move calcium into the bones, while suppressing the release of parathyroid hormone (PTH) that draws calcium out of the bones, depositing it in soft tissue. Calcium, when taken alone, does not suppress the release of PTH, according to the authors.

The alternative approach suggests that hardness of the bone is only half of the story. The other half is in the protein matrix of the bone that creates bone flexibility. Flexible bones are harder to break. Magnesium helps create bone flexibility. They also advise that vitamin D and trace boron help calcium and magnesium work better together.

Bodmer and Fuchs also relate the findings of well-known California research gynecologist and endocrinologist, Guy E. Abraham, M.D., who advises his patients take from 200 to 1000 mg. of magnesium per day to build bone strength. "These women showed an average bone density increase of 11 percent in one year, by adjusting their diets to increase magnesium (500-1000 mg/day) and lower calcium (500 mg/day)," write the authors.

For we chocoholics, the authors believe our chocolate cravings may be from an imbalance of calcium/magnesium. They state that cocoa powder contains more magnesium than any other food; hence, our bodies may be craving the magnesium we need. When we add sugar and butter to chocolate, we lose all benefits because high sugar intake causes magnesium excretion as well as calcium loss. They believe that if we eat more green vegetables, lentils, split peas and other legumes and avoid sugars and sodas, our cravings will be suppressed due to sufficient magnesium/calcium ratio. I believe that suggests my Friday trip to Fannie May Candies "for old times' sake" was not a very good idea. Downright depressing.

I am presently gathering information on several promising studies showing that another natural element, strontium may also be helpful in building bone mass.

CHLORELLA—WONDER FOOD FOR DIGESTION, IMMUNE FUNCTION AND HEAVY METAL REMOVAL

Very often we read about "wonder" foods always remembering to take the claims with a grain of salt. Because I read so much on health and try many products, I have personally learned that many claims are quite exaggerated. Scientific research must become part of the quotient when determining the validity of such claims. Most recently, when I gathered research on a product known as "chlorella" I learned that it is probably one of the most scientifically studied foods on the planet. It can easily be considered a near perfect food. It's an algae product with very high chlorophyll content as well as nutrients and enzymes. Chlorella is not a supplement or vitamin. It is considered a whole food product, however, it contains unique fiber, vitamins, enzymes and even chlorophyll. In fact, it contains more chlorophyll per gram than any other food product.

Among the many functions of chlorella is its ability to bind to heavy metals washing them out of the body through the elimination process. Dr. Joseph Mercola writes about the wonders of chlorella, a rich green food that feeds and detoxifies the body as no other. According to Mercola, "Numerous research projects in the USA and Europe indicate that chlorella can also aid the body in the breakdown of persistent hydrocarbon and metallic toxins such as DDT, PCB, mercury, cadmium and lead, while strengthening the immune system response. In Japan, interest in chlorella has focused largely on its detoxifying properties—its ability to neutralize or remove poisonous substances from the body." According to the literature, chlorella affects the removal of these substances over a period of three to six months.

The indigestible fibrous outer shell of chlorella is what helps bind it to toxins and wash them from the body. Alternative physicians consider chlorella a cleanser as well as a tonic and immune supporter.

Dr. Mercola writes of chlorella's benefits to the digestive tract as well as its cleansing and immune building properties. Chlorella creates an intestinal environment that allows the friendly bacteria that our bodies need, to replicate faster. In addition to containing chlorophyll, chlorella contains the digestive enzymes chlorophyllase and pepsin, both enzymes help process our foods while gleaning the nutrients from foods we eat. Mercola advises that the best chlorella is not pasteurized or freeze-dried. He states the enzymes are destroyed through such processes. According to Mercola, it takes between three to five months of regular normal dosage to work effectively, however, he states, you should feel other signs of improvement a bit earlier. He describes digestion as being quickly aided by chlorella and reports: "The first thing is better digestion, especially if you have bad breath or constipation. Both these are readily handled by taking small doses of Chlorella. However, many of the benefits of chlorella are subtle and not easily determined by how a person feels." There are numerous additional benefits in taking the right form of chlorella on a regular basis. An important aspect of natural foods and natural healing is that there is a time element involved. Sometimes it takes weeks and months to feel the difference. Patience and perseverance will pay off. It's always easier to take a quick-fix pill that may mask the symptoms, but getting to the root of the problem and correcting bad habits, will always prove more rewarding.

For instance, Chlorella has been demonstrated to remove heavy metals and other synthetics from the body by actually binding with them so they may be pulled from the bloodstream. However, this result can only be measured if the level of heavy metals in the bloodstream is known before and after a person starts taking chlorella.

According to literature, it takes approximately 3-6 months once starting chlorella for heavy metals to begin clearing from the blood depending on the amount of chlorella taken. If it has been determined that a person does have heavy metals in their body, they should begin by taking 15-20 grams per day depending on the level of heavy metals that are present. according to Dr. Joseph Mercola. *Also see MCP and DMPS for heavy metal removal*

CHOLESTEROL: A SPECIAL TEST YOU NEED

Do you think you're getting the latest, most accurate cholesterol blood test available? Chances are you're not. The next time your doctor orders cholesterol testing, suggest he/she include a newer test that breaks down your cholesterol into even smaller and more accurate markers of possible health and heart problems in the future.

As you may already know, simple total cholesterol testing is not an effective measure of artery or heart condition. Fifty percent of heart attacks occur among people with normal total cholesterol levels.

You may also be aware that measuring HDL (high density lipoprotein) against LDL (low density lipoprotein) has gained some momentum in the health community. HDL is your good cholesterol. The higher the number, the better. LDL is considered your "bad" cholesterol. The lower the number, the better. This is not always the case with LDL.

A newer discovery is showing that LDL cholesterol is not all bad. The newer discovery has shown that there are also "good" and "bad" components within your LDL cholesterol itself. LDL cholesterol contains both large and small particles. The larger particles have been shown to repair artery damage and wash out of the system. This is the good part of your LDL cholesterol. These particles are also contained in your HDL cholesterol. It's part of what makes HDL so good. These larger particles are doing exactly what cholesterol was meant to do—repair damage. On the other hand, LDL contains smaller particles that can remain within the arteries without easily washing out. The smaller particles can pack in along arteries and create hardening of the arteries and other vascular problems.

I first saw the new test referenced in Dr. Robert Jay Rowen's *Second Opinion* newsletter. I then researched to get further documentation on the information he covered. The new test was discussed at the annual meeting of the European Society of Cardiology in September of 2004. Rowen explained that the large particles known as apolipoprotein A1 (apo A1) are your "good" LDL cholesterol components while the smaller particles known as apolipoprotein B (apo B) were the troublesome factor in your LDL.

Dr. Salim Yusef, professor of medicine at McMaster University in Canada was quoted as having stated, "50% of the risk of a heart attack is predicted by the apo B/apo A1 ratio."

The simple test measures the number of large and small particles in your LDL cholesterol and then measures a ratio to determine your risk factors. By using the apo B/apo A1 test, doctors were said to be able to attain a far more predictive and accurate picture of where your heart and arteries are headed in the future. A ratio of 1 to 1 is considered high risk. A ratio where you have more small than large particles indicates an even higher risk.

The new test is said to be a simple test and the blood can be drawn before or after a meal with no fasting required. You may want to ask your physician to order an apo B/apo A1.

It was suggested at the conference that many physicians might take a while to accept and order the new tests. You can be the first on your block to learn about your risk factors based on these two fractions of your LDL. Go for it.

CHOLESTEROL HIGH? FIGHT IT WITH POLICOSANOL

There's a remarkable natural substance made from a fraction of sugar cane that can lower your cholesterol, triglycerides, blood pressure, help prevent platelet aggregation (clotting) does not deplete your body of Coenzyme Q10, (a most necessary nutrient), yet, you most likely have never heard of it. It's derived from a fraction of the sugar cane, yet it will not affect your blood sugar levels. It cannot be patented as a drug, has virtually no-side effects, and costs less than one-half the price of dangerous statin drugs which are used to reduce cholesterol. It can actually help your body produce more HDL (good cholesterol), according to Robert Rowen, M.D. He says HDL is the cholesterol that helps your body fight plaque build up in your arteries. The substance is known as policosanol and you can purchase it at any health food store. There are no big bucks in the sale of policosanol products, so don't expect to hear about it in the mainstream media or medical community.

According to another of the alternative community's top physicians, Dr. Jonathan Wright, policosanol was tested against the commonly used statin drugs in randomized, double-blind, placebo-controlled studies. It was first tested among individuals with type 2 diabetes and high cholesterol. All individuals followed a lipid-lowering diet for six weeks. They were then divided into two groups. One group was given 20 milligrams of Mevacor (a statin drug) daily, while the other was given 10 milligrams of policosanol daily for 12 weeks. Both groups experienced lowered total cholesterol, but the policosanol group's bad cholesterol, (LDL) was decreased by 4 percent more than the Mevacor group. The good cholesterol level (HDL) rose nearly 8 percent compared to a 3 percent drop in the Mevacor group. When it came to measurement of the triglycerides, there was no question policosanol was superior. Policosanol caused an 18 percent drop in triglycerides, while Mevacor dropped the triglycerides by only 0.5 percent.

Policosanol was also found to drop the systolic (top number) blood pressure by 8 points and the diastolic (lower number) was reduced by approximately three points. Mevacor, on the other hand, increased the blood pressure by several points.

Dr. Wright published additional study results which pitted policosanol against Zocor among "53 individuals ages 60 to 77 with "primary hypercholesterolemia" (high cholesterol not linked to diabetes or other known metabolic problems)." Once again, one of the groups took 10 mg. of policosanol daily while the other took 10 mg. of Zocor. Both groups reduced overall cholesterol levels, but the policosanol group showed 5 percent lower triglyceride levels.

In an even more astonishing outcome, when policosanol was tested against the popular statin drug, Pravachol, there was no race. Policosanol worked better. It lowered the (LDL) bad cholesterol levels and reduced triglycerides 11 percent more than Pravachol while raising the good cholesterol levels by 18 percent more than Pravachol, according to Dr. Wright.

So what else is good about policosanol, aside from cost, effectiveness and its ability to reduce stroke risks by inhibiting platelet aggregation better than any of the statin drugs? It's good for you, says Dr. Wright, unlike statin drugs that can destroy your liver and muscles. Additionally, there is now a new question as to the relationship between cholesterol lowering drugs and an increase in peripheral neuropathy among those taking statins.

Don't you ever wonder why you have probably never heard of policosanol? Why not ask your doctor if he or she has heard about policosanol. I'll bet they are in the dark as much as most other Americans. Doesn't this make you wonder about what is happening in conventional medicine?

Senior citizens should not be asking for free medicines, they should be asking why safe, less expensive, alternatives are not being made available to them. The fact is, as we age, our liver loses its ability to process many things, including medications, especially harsh medications that can create both liver problems and muscle break-down. That's why patients prescribed many prescription drugs must obtain regular blood tests to assure there has been no harm to the liver, muscles and other organs.

If the government and medical community, Medicare, HMO's and PPO's were to insist that the less expensive, but equally effective alternatives be used, health costs in the United States would be reduced and you would be a great deal safer. But with the amount of money made on patented drugs, don't count on too many positive changes in the system.

There is good science behind this wonder pill. Studies have shown it to be as effective and in some cases, more effective than some of the statin drugs. In the case of Pravachol, the randomized double blind, placebo controlled studies showed policosanol to be far superior to Pravachol. When it comes to reducing triglycerides, it's the best. It's about one-half the price of any statin drug, and if you purchase it from vitamin outlet stores, you can obtain even better prices. Policosanol does not interfere with liver function or cause liver damage as many of the statin drugs can. It also does not reduce the body's stores of Coenzyme Ql0 (CoQ10) as do the statin drugs. It decreases LDL (bad cholesterol) levels and increases the HDL, (good cholesterol) levels. So far its greatest function appears to be in reducing triglycerides. The best part of using policosanol, is that it has no side effects.

More recent studies have found it to be helpful in slightly reducing blood pressure as well. In the original study, Mevacor slightly increased blood pressure while policosanol slightly reduced blood pressure. I have also read of another study that shows it to be helpful against a condition known as intermittent claudication, a circulatory disorder that makes walking very difficult for many patients who suffer leg cramps or pain after walking only short distances.

The reason most have never heard of policosanol or seen the studies of its effectiveness are because it is a natural substance that cannot be patented. When pharmaceutical companies are unable to patent a product, that product will not produce market shares and cannot reap millions for pharmaceuticals. That is part of why we need to understand that conventional health care is dangerously cluttered by money and politics. For that reason I enjoy reporting on such natural and healthy methods for solving health problems.

One of the observations I have made in reading about both the statins and policosanol is that with more wide-based usage of policosanol, additional health benefits are being discovered. That is not the case with most pharmaceuticals. In fact, many times after broad-based usage, they are discovered to have even more side-effects than originally considered.

Recently, I received a phone call from a friend who excitedly read his new blood test results to me after having taken policosanol for over six months. His blood tests showed his outrageously high triglycerides had dropped more than 200 points and his total cholesterol had also been greatly reduced. I appreciate it when others share their test results with me.

As always, discuss these matters with your family physician because policosanol, if taken with a statin, may reduce cholesterol much more than desired. The dosage used in the tests was 20 mg. per day. Just a note: How many of those taking statin drugs have been told by their physicians that statins are one of the many drugs that deplete the body of Coenzyme Q10 and that the coenzyme Q10 must be replaced?

Further studies have shown that the only really effective policosanol is that which is derived from sugar cane, the most potent being Cuban sugar cane.

COENZYME Q10—HEART AND CELLULAR ENERGY

I pored over literature and studies related to newer information on Coenzyme Q10 (CoQ10,) also known as Ubiquinone. Many alternative physicians are concerned that certain classes of drugs deplete the body's stores of this essential coenzyme found in the muscle cell mitochondria, responsible for enzyme activity associated with the production of energy. One of the major CoQ10 depleting culprits are statin drugs for lowering cholesterol. The medical establishment is slowly recognizing the need for adjunctive supplementation with CoQ10 among statin drug users,—perhaps while Rome burns. The Food & Drug Administration (FDA) prefers to "reserve judgment" on CoQ10 augmentation. Coenzyme Q10 cannot be patented. It is natural.

Many conventional physicians are puzzled by the rise in cardiomyopathy (heart failure) in spite of the numerous advances in medical technology. The question may be: Can some cardiomyopathy be related to the ever-increasing usage of cholesterol lowering drugs because they deplete CoQ10? Note that cholesterol-lowering drugs have now exceeded blood pressure medications in profits for pharmaceuticals. There is urgency here. These statins were once dispensed to about 13,000,000 patients, however, since the new lower cholesterol guidelines have been adopted, up to 36,000,000 patients may be candidates for these drugs. None of these drugs carry the warning about depletion of CoQ10. That is, unless you purchase your statins from Canadian pharmaceuticals. Canada requires warnings on statins explaining they may deplete CoQ10.

An article by Kurt J Samson, appearing in the August, 2004 issue of "*Life Extension Magazine*" discusses many of the promising results found in clinical trials pertaining to the use of CoQ10 for numerous disorders. Among the results he lists are studies showing that in small clinical trials of kidney failure patients, CoQ10 increased the kidney's ability to rid the body of toxic wastes. In one 12-week study, patients with end-stage renal failure were given CoQ10 as well as their other conventional therapies, and many of the patients were found to have decreased progression and even reversal of renal dysfunction, with some patients not even requiring dialysis during the 12-week study. According to the editors of *Life Extension*, newer studies indicate we lose our natural stores of CoQ10 much more rapidly than once believed. The studies also indicate that larger amounts than 30 mg. per day of CoQ10 are needed and can be taken for better results.

Coenzyme Q10 is so pivotal to health that Dr. Stephen Sinatra of the New England Heart Clinic, goes on record as stating that if his patients had a choice of taking only one supplement, it would be CoQ10.

Alternative physicians believe that CoQ10 absolutely must be added to the regimen of all patients taking statin drugs, such as, Mevacor, Lipitor, Pravachol and Zocor as well as some other medications. They note that even aspirin depletes CoQ10 supplies. This essential coenzyme supplies the cells with energy and acts as a cell nutrient and provides cardiac strength, according to Stephen Sinatra, M.D. He stated that he now prescribes heart-healthy CoQ10 to all of his heart patients with special emphasis on those taking statin drugs.

It is no wonder that such a helpful, natural occurring enzyme might also be discovered to possess broad applications in alleviating other disorders.

Coenzyme Q10 slows Parkinson's progression

Most recently, studies have shown that Coenzyme Q10 seems to be helpful in reducing the progression of Parkinson's disease, according to Dr. Jonathan Wright. Wright explains that researchers from around the U.S. teamed up to identify therapies that may be helpful in treating Parkinsonism. The results of the study which appeared recently in the Archives of Neurology, indicated that early-stage Parkinson's patients were helped by the administration of coenzyme Q10. Three of the four groups were given varying dosages of coenzyme Q10, with the control group given placebo. All patients in the three coenzyme Q10 groups showed improvement in the form of a decrease in the rate of functional decline, with the largest improvement seen in the group taking the highest dose of CoQ10. Researchers are now planning even larger trials with higher doses of CoQ10. The actual abstract as posted on PUB/MED read: "CONCLUSIONS: Coenzyme Q10 was safe and well tolerated at dosages of up to 1200 mg./d. Less disability developed in subjects assigned to coenzyme Q10 than in those assigned to placebo, and the benefit was greatest in subjects receiving the highest dosage. Coenzyme Q10 appears to slow the progressive deterioration of function in PD, but these results need to be confirmed in a larger study." I might add that average dosage ranges from 30 mg. to 200 mg. and the dosage of 1200 should never be taken by anyone without being prescribed by a physician or as a part of a closely monitored study.

Potential use in muscular disorders

Dr. Sinatra, who was one of the first to discover the benefits of augmentation with CoQ10, also believes the essential energy enzyme will be useful in treating many other diseases, including numerous muscular-related disorders. Sinatra points out that "The late Dr. Karl Folkers, who is the acknowledged father of CoQ10, concluded that anyone suffering from muscular dystrophy, or for that matter, any mitochondrial disorder, should be treated with CoQ10 indefinitely." Sinatra states that early studies indicate it improves quality of life for those suffering such ravaging diseases. Sinatra sees it as being a potential help in the treatment of Muscular Dystrophy, Lou Gehrig's Disease (ALS), Multiple Sclerosis and many other muscular disorders.

Alternative physician, Joseph Mercola says: "While I am not a great fan of using supplements as Band-Aids, by the time someone has Parkinson's disease the horse is already out of the barn, and coenzyme Q10 appears to be a useful supplement. CoQ10 is normally made by the liver and is decreased when someone is placed on statin drugs. A prescription for lipid lowering statin drugs should always be accompanied with a recommendation to take CoQ10, because if one is deficient in it (CoQ10) heart failure is more likely."

Dr. Mercola also feels that CoQ10 is also helpful when used as an adjunct to cancer therapy. His reasoning is that it protects the heart from cardiotoxicity caused by anthracycline chemotherapy drugs that also have the potential for creating heart damage.

The enzyme was first discovered in 1957. Studies in Sweden and the U.S. that go back as far as 1961 showed a CoQ10 deficiency among cancer patients, especially in cases of those with diagnosed breast cancer.

Dr. Mercola's website has a great deal of information on the studies of CoQ10 and its use in cancer treatment and therapy.

Mercola lists a source for more information on complementary and alternative therapies as the NIH National Center for Complementary and Alternative Medicine (NCCAM), NCCAM Clearinghouse, P.O. Box 8218, Silver Springs, Md. 20907-0210. A new super-absorbable CoQ10 can be purchased at Life Extension Foundation (800-544-4440)

COENZYME Q10 AS AN ADJUNCT TO STATIN DRUGS

If your doctor suggests that the jury is still out when it comes to using CoQ10 as an adjunctive therapy to your statin drug prescription, you may want to ask your doctor why pharmaceutical "inventors" from Merck & Co. (maker of Zocor) were assigned two most interesting patents that allows them to add CoQ10 directly to statin drugs in the manufacturing process. Yes, Merck states in their patent application that adding CoQ10 to their statins may not only prevent myopathies, but it will reduce chances of sustaining liver damage.

Statin drugs are known technically as HMG-CoA reductase inhibitors. I conducted a search of the U.S. Patent Office and found patent #4,929,437 and 4,933,165 awarded to Merck, along with an abstract addressing the issue in medical terminology: "Abstract: A pharmaceutical composition and method of counteracting HMG-CoA reductase inhibitor-associated myopathy is disclosed. The method comprises the adjunct administration of an effective amount of an HMG-CoA reductase inhibitor and an effective amount of Coenzyme Q sub 10." In essence, they want to manufacture the statins along with the necessary CoQ10 to avoid myopathies. Claim #3 on the Merck patent states: 3. A method of counteracting HMG-CoA reductase inhibitor-associated skeletal muscle myopathy in a subject in need of such treatment which comprises the adjunct administration of a therapeutically effective amount of an HMG-CoA reductase inhibitor and an effective amount of Coenzyme Q.sub.10 to counteract said myopathy." They further state CoQ10 will help fight liver damage caused by statins.

So what happened? Why did this company obtain these patents if they didn't want to use them? Perhaps, adding CoQ10 would cut profit margins? Even though conventional medicine is slow in catching on about the importance of CoQ10, it might be wise for those taking statins to bring the information on the patents to their physicians for explanations. According to a *Life Extension* article, several studies by respected researchers warned of the problems of CoQ10 depletion at the very time Pfizer Pharmaceuticals placed Lipitor on the market.

Coenzyme Q10 is good for the heart, but it's also proving exceptionally useful in supporting other organs and other conditions, not only based on the fact that it is an enzyme responsible for the creation of cellular energy, but also based on well-designed studies. Several exciting studies were referenced in *Life Extension Magazine*, August 2004. One reference involved a randomized, double blind, placebo controlled 12-week study on adjunctive therapy in which 180 mg. of CoQ10 was administered to patients with end-stage kidney failure. The results indicated that only one-half of the kidney patients required dialysis during the 12 week period. The CoQ10 reduced the levels of serum creatinine and blood urea nitrogen and increased urine output. The article goes on to explain that renal function was improved regardless of dialysis status. This study also concluded that other plasma poisoning substances, fell dramatically among those administered the CoQ10. The researchers suggested that higher doses than 180 mg. might show even more positive results.

In yet another study, patients with muscular dystrophy who received CoQ10 therapy showed "significantly less cytogenic and DNA damage than their untreated counterparts, according to a study by Dr. Lucia Migliore and colleagues at Pisa University in Italy."

The *Life Extension* article also related the results of several studies on patients with prostate cancer. The studies indicated "CoQ10 supplementation significantly lowered cell growth of the PC3 cancer line without affecting non-malignant cells." In even further studies a deficiency of CoQ10 was found in the brains of 17 patients with cerebellar ataxia (defective coordination) and/or atrophy (wasting away).

DIABETES—BENFOTIAMINE: THIAMINE DERIVATIVE SHOWS RESULTS

As I pored over information on anti-aging, I came across what appears to be the latest breakthrough on fighting diabetes and diabetic neuropathy as well as retinopathy. The substance is known as benfotiamine, derived from the B-vitamin thiamine (B-1).

The process used to create benfotiamine was patented in Japan in 1962, and benfotiamine has been used successfully in Europe for over 10 years to relieve diabetic neuropathies. Unlike regular B-vitamins that are water soluble, benfotiamine is fat-soluble which means the body can store up enough to be effective. Water-soluble vitamins are transient and that which is not utilized wash out or pass through our bodies without being stored up in a cumulative fashion. Our bodies absorb all nutrients based on the ability to assimilate whatever vitamins are ingested. Sometimes vitamins are made so inexpensively that they do not go through the digestive process. They exit the body in the same condition as they entered.

As we age we become less able to assimilate both foods and vitamins; hence, many water soluble vitamins merely wash out or pass through our digestive system unless we have adequate digestive enzymes and stomach acid. The quality of our absorption declines with age because the quality of our digestive system and enzyme capacity steadily decreases with age.

In the case of fat-soluble vitamins, such as vitamin E and vitamin A, they are not easily eliminated. In fact, vitamin A can be toxic if too much is ingested because it can accumulate in the system.

Once again, according to *Life Extension Magazine,* January 2004, benfotiamine not only shows promise in controlling neuropathy, but it is helpful with controlling a number of disease processes including diabetes itself.

The magazine reports, "Recently, scientists have begun taking a closer look at benfotiamine, a compound derived from thiamine. Used for more than a decade in Germany to treat nerve pain in diabetics, benfotiamine is fat soluble and therefore considerably more available to the body than thiamine.

A landmark new study, published earlier this year in the medical journal *Nature Medicine,* found that benfotiamine increases transketolase activity in cell cultures by an astounding 300%. By comparison, when thiamine was added to cell cultures, transketolase activity increased a mere 20%. This robust activation of transketolase by benfotiamine was sufficient to block three of the four major metabolic pathways leading to blood vessel damage. Additionally, benfotiamine blocked activation of the pro-inflammatory transcription factor NF-kB. This suggests yet another beneficial attribute of benfotiamine." In essence, the article explains that benfotiamine provides numerous positive health functions in addition to its promise for diabetes.

Benfotiamine demonstrated that it prevents damage to blood vessel cells in test tube experiments. It also helped prevent retinal damage in animal testing. The bulk of the testing in the U.S. has been on animals, even though it has been used successfully in Europe. Larger human studies were conducted in Bulgaria with positive results and larger human trials in this country will become necessary before it is approved by the Food & Drug Administration (FDA).

DIGESTION—ENZYMES ARE ESSENTIAL TO GOOD HEALTH

Proper digestion is just as important as diet and that requires enzymes. Raw foods contain the necessary enzymes that explain why alternative physicians suggest the bulk of our diets contain raw vegetables and fruits. Enzymes serve to properly break down fats, proteins, starches, carbs and sugars. If they are not adequately broken down, where do you suppose they go? They form fat deposits while our bodies basically starve for the nutrients that many times pass right through our bodies un-digested.

Digestive problems comprise the number one health issue on the North American continent. The treatment of digestive disorders within the conventional medical community is an area of contention among conventional and alternative physicians. Millions of Americans are taking antacids that do nothing more than treat and mask symptoms. There is little understanding of the essential role enzymes and acids play in facilitating the digestive process that keep our bodies in balance and well fed. Alternative physicians believe one must take the time to seek out the causes of indigestion and address those causes rather than merely treat symptoms. Generally speaking, conventional medicine treats indigestion with pills because pills seem to eliminate the symptoms.

Alternative physicians believe that masking symptoms is dangerous because the negative conditions that created the disorder in the first place, continue to inflict damage to the system, even in the absence of symptoms. An example I recently covered was related to gastroesophageal reflux disorder (GERD). Some of the medication circulars quietly advise that harm to the esophagus may continue even while the medications may resolve the symptoms. How can such danger be so easily overlooked?

It's important to realize that digestion is the process by which we fuel our bodies. Enzymes are abundantly available in raw foods. When we eat processed foods, such as some of the high-fat burgers, our bodies struggle with both the lack of enzymes and the high fat content which is even harder to digest and may end up in our arteries as well as our backsides. It's also important for each of us to understand that as we age, our digestive enzymes are harder to come by. We generally do very well with enzymes and metabolism until we reach the tender age of 25. After that, many of us begin to reduce our metabolic function.

One exceptional digestive enzyme is bromelain, derived from pineapple stems. Bromelain is one of several enzymes that help repair muscle and tissue. Bromelain also possesses anti-inflammatory properties as well. In turn, these anti-inflammatory constituents also serve as a natural inhibitor of platelet aggregation that can result in blood clots. So you can see there is a cycle that helps establish good health.

Since most of us eat cooked and microwaved foods, supplementation with enzymes is more than just a good idea. The alternative stance is that if you eat many processed foods, you should always supplement with proper digestive enzymes. Remember, enzymes and acids are the foundation of the entire digestive cycle.

DRUG INTERACTIONS—DO NOT MIX AND MATCH

The nutritional and healing effects of various herb and food constituents, roots and leaves—even common juices, can have a negative effect when taken with various drugs and even foods. The most common example of drug interactions involves grapefruit juice. Grapefruit is delicious and grapefruits are chock full of vitamins as well as other great nutrients including bioflavonoids and fiber, however; when grapefruit juice is taken with certain medicines, or even with something as simple as a cup of coffee, it can cause severe reactions. Yes, caffeine and grapefruit juice taken at the same time can prove dangerous.

In June of 2002, the publishers of Worst Pills/Best Pills listed various drug interactions that occur when grapefruit juice is consumed along with various drugs. Among the drugs that create the worst reactions are statins (Lipitor, Zocor, Pravachol) etc. Other serious reactions can occur if BuSpar or Tegretol are taken with grapefruit juice. There are many milder to moderate reactions when taken with other drugs, so it's probably best not to take any medications with grapefruit juice, just to be on the safe side. That doesn't mean everyone should give up grapefruit. Eat it at another time of the day because it's healthy.

In "The People's Pharmacy Guide to Home and Herbal Remedies" the authors list several other dangerous combinations of drugs. They explain that one should not take drugs such as Coumadin along with Gingko. Gingko is believed to stimulate blood flow, which is why it is touted as brain food. Gingko should not be taken when a patient is taking any type of blood thinners.

Kava should not be taken when one is taking the anti-anxiety drug, Xanax (Alprazolam), or numerous other anti-anxiety drugs such as Valium, Librium, Ativan or Dalmane. Kava is a mainstay beverage in the Fiji Islands, which may explain why the islanders are so mellow—according to my son and daughter-in-law who recently visited the islands.

Another interesting herb is St. John's Wort, an excellent natural relaxing herb that should never be taken concomitantly with Paxil or any other antidepressant. St. John's Wort is also what is known as a very mild MAO (monoamine oxidase—a chemical associated with depression) inhibitor, which means certain foods may interact with it. Among those foods to avoid when taking St. John's Wort, is vinegar, cheeses and smoked foods. The Food & Drug Administration (FDA) issued an advisory that St. John's Wort interfered with the effectiveness of the HIV drug Indinavir.

The authors also explain that licorice used on a regular basis should not be mixed with Lanoxin because licorice over time can reduce with the body's potassium levels. If licorice is taken regularly along with Lanoxin, potassium levels could become dangerously low.

Interactions are even more common when a patient is taking more than six drugs. I found information worth noting on the web site of Dr. Joseph Mercola. "Statistically, if you take six different drugs, you have an 80 percent chance of at least one drug-drug interaction. With eight drugs, the chance is 100 percent." The statement is attributed to Wayne K. Anderson, dean of the School of Pharmacy and Pharmaceutical Sciences at the State University of New York at Buffalo.

Our new drug or "drugged" culture makes interactions more likely. Even more unfortunately, there is a great effort being expended to direct many drugs that modify brain chemistry in our children and our grandchildren. The word "unconscionable" comes to mind, but I would bet, given the proper spin, more children will become targets of the pharmaceuticals. Watch for those interactions and always remember that diet affects every aspect of our very being and many of the disorders we suffer are related to nutritional deficiencies, not to pharmaceutical deficiencies!

DRUGS THAT DEPLETE NUTRIENTS

There comes a time in most lifetimes when prescription drugs may be needed. Hopefully, on a temporary basis, but sometimes long term. One of the problems with many pharmaceuticals is that they can deplete our systems of necessary nutrients and sometimes block absorption of various additional essential nutrients. This depletion can actually make us feel worse, especially when drugs are taken over long periods of time.

Cholesterol reducing drugs also deplete melatonin, a hormone that helps accommodate sleep.

We can mitigate the collateral damage of some drugs by supplementing with the depleted nutrients. Perhaps those who were unaware of the problems associated with prolonged drug therapy may wish to consult their physicians regarding the efficacy of supplementation with corresponding depleted nutrients. Those supplementations, in many cases, may actually enhance the medication's effectiveness.

Drugs that deplete

Aspirin, acid blockers, (Tagamet, Pepcid, Zantac, Prevacid) and certain cholesterol-lowering medications such as Questran, can deplete your body of iron. It may take four to six months for the first signs of anemia (fatigue, weakness, hair loss) to appear. It may take some time for your doctor to suspect or diagnose iron-deficiency anemia, according to "Alternatives" newsletter.

Drugs that deplete B-Vitamins, Coenzyme Q10, and Zinc

Estrogen-containing drugs are known to cause deficiencies of many important nutrients, including vitamin B6, Vitamin B-12, folic acid and Vitamin F (unsaturated fatty acids). They also can deplete amino acids. Birth-control pills are among those estrogen containing drugs that reduce B-Vitamins. Women taking birth-control pills may want to supplement with B-complex. Anxiety or depression can be signs of B-vitamin deficiency. Antibiotics deplete vitamin B and vitamin K as well as the friendly bacteria in the intestines and colon.

The prescription drug, Prilosec reduces Bl2 levels. "Prilosec decreases intrinsic factor which is the chemical needed by the body to absorb vitamin Bl2," according to Dr. David Williams' "Alternative Newsletter."

Beta-blockers (heart and blood pressure drug) reduce Coenzyme Ql0, as do statin drugs. Anti-viral agents, steroids, oral contraceptives and estrogens, along with ACE Inhibitors (another type of blood pressure drugs) and diuretics also decrease the body's supply of zinc and Coenzyme Ql0. Psychotherapeutic medications can cause B6 and Coenzyme Ql0 deficiencies as well.

OTHER DRUG DEPLETIONS

Anti-inflammatory drugs deplete minerals, Vitamin C, D and F (unsaturated fatty acids). Even some of the foods we eat that are high in sugars can deplete other essential nutrients.

These are only a few of the many drugs that deplete, so if you are on long term drugs, you may wish to purchase the book, "Drug-Induced Nutrient Depletion Handbook", (Lexi-Comp Clinical Reference Library, 1999). It addresses nearly 1,000 drugs that can cause nutrient depletion. It also contains comprehensive citations and abstracts from the actual medical literature. For information or to order the book call Lexi-Comp at: 800-837-5394 or 330-650-6506.

EAT FOR YOUR BLOOD TYPE

Your blood type can determine your physical weaknesses and your special nutritional and physical needs, according to Peter D'Adamo, author of "Eat (4) for your Blood Type." Dr. D'Adamo claims we all have biochemical individuality, which makes us both sensitive and responsive to numerous foods based on our blood types.

According to D'Adamo, our individual blood type is like a genetic fingerprint, carrying genetic strengths and weaknesses. D'Adamo lists the four blood types (A, B, AB, O) along with the particular foods that will cause weight gain in those blood types as well as the foods that will enhance weight loss in specific types. But even more significant is his breakdown of foods that he believes are essential to promote good health in each blood type.

D'Adamo explains that certain blood types react better to certain foods and that some blood types should avoid other specific foods that we may ingest on a daily basis. The book is an easy read, especially if we just focus on the information he compiles addressing our individual blood type. An interesting aspect of his theory is that, according to D'Adamo, some foods that we all consider beneficial are not equally beneficial to all blood types and can be more difficult for one blood type to digest than another blood type. The information and explanations are very detailed for each blood type. As an example, blood type A's do not handle meat well, and are better suited to a vegetarian-type diet, according to Dr. D'Adamo, while blood type O's are born carnivores and need meat. He states that each blood type has strengths and weaknesses that should be addressed through diet and lifestyle changes.

D'Adamo even lists which vitamin supplements are most needed by each blood type. He also posits that blood type A's will have fewer reactions to vaccinations than other blood types, but type A's will also be more prone to infections.

Based on individual blood types, he even prescribes which types of exercise that would be most beneficial for each blood type. Type A's need less rigorous exercises such as yoga and Tai Chi while O's should perform more aerobics and participate in the more vigorous workouts. Type B should have moderate workouts, and AB's need calming exercises and should participate in more relaxation stretches.

He includes a chapter on herbs for various conditions as well as herbs that certain blood types should avoid.

Since my blood type is A, of course, that was my first chapter. I was astonished at the accuracy of D'Adamo's statements pertaining to my own experience with foods. I have already lived the experience and am pretty well aware of problems with certain foods and was surprised to see those foods listed in his book under my blood type. If his rationalizations are correct, they would seem to help explain why some people appear to handle certain conditions better than others and why some people eating the same foods and living the same basic lives develop particular diseases while others seem to remain healthy. There are usually many factors that contribute to one's propensity toward disease, such as genetics, environmental factors and attitude, (attitude being a major factor) but D'Adamo's theory may prove to be quite helpful when assessing the overall picture.

The manner in which our bodies tolerate and digest what we feed them, is certainly essential to overall health. The exception to the rule will show up here and there, but generally speaking, there appears to be growing acceptance of his research.

Dr. D'Adamo has worked with numerous other physicians in addressing disease, wellness and general health, based on blood typing. One of his first admirers has been alternative physician, Jonathan Wright, M.D. Is this book just a fad or another important piece to the puzzle? Whether medical science views him as a heretic or an Einstein, will remain to be seen, but in the meantime, we patients should consider that there was a time when Pasteur was ridiculed by "Modern Science" and just 10 years ago, researchers who claimed that inflammation was involved in heart disease, were castaways.

The background for the book was a result of the impressions of Peter's father, James D'Adamo, a naturopathic physician, who noticed that while many of his patients did very well on a low-fat, strict vegetarian diets, some became worse and were unable to handle a vegetarian diet. A one-size-fits-all approach to health or most anything else in life, will rarely work because we all function as individuals.

While we have some common profiles in basic human behavior, we react differently to various circumstances. D'Adamo's father, operated on the basis of the old adage that "one man's poison is another man's meat" as he proceeded to look for answers to why there were such variances in reactions to diets. He felt there must be some type of blueprint, which would account for the difference in reactions to the diets. His patients who fared poorly on strict vegetarian diets were those with type O blood. They seemed to thrive on meat, much better than any of the other blood types. The elder D'Adamo noticed that those patients who could handle the vegetarian diet best were those with type A blood. He also noticed conversely, patients with type A blood, attempting to utilize meat as their main protein source, did not fare well at all; however, when put on vegetable forms of protein and legumes, they flourished. In 1980 the senior D'Adamo authored a book, *One Man's Food* explaining his theories about food tolerance and blood types.

Another observation of the elder D'Adamo was that vigorous exercise did not suit all patients. Again, he found that those with type A blood did not do well with vigorous exercise, while those with blood type O handled vigorous exercise very well. Blood type A, he says, is more suited toward Tai Chi, Yoga and light weight lifting.

A young Peter D'Adamo, while in his senior year at Bastyr College, decided to take his father's theory one step further to see if his father's subjective impressions carried any scientific weight. He determined to seek more objective methods of verifying the blood type theory. D'Adamo scanned medical literature and found his first breakthrough when he says he discovered that two major diseases of the stomach were associated with blood type. The first was the peptic ulcer, a condition often related to higher than average stomach-acid levels in those with type O blood. "This condition was reported to be more common in people with type O blood than in other blood types," D'Adamo wrote. To D'Adamo, this would explain why type O's seemed to possess the ability to handle and digest meats better than type A's. On the other hand D'Adamo found more stomach cancers in blood type A's. According to D'Adamo, blood type A's have less stomach acid production. He found the same to be the case with many patients suffering pernicious anemia, which is related to lack of vitamin B-12 absorption that requires sufficient stomach acid.

His next step was to prove that various foods affected the actual health of patients whose blood types did not agree with those foods. The culprits, according to D'Adamo, are known as "lectins," sticky, agglutinating proteins in food; which can be shown to affect one blood type more than others. Lectin activity, according to D'Adamo, can be measured from a urine specimen, to assess intestinal conditions that lead to immune problems by causing cells to clump together—a dangerous process, according to D'Adamo.

Very simply put, his theory is that when we eat the wrong foods for our blood type, the foods act to cause our immune systems to react as if we were fighting a disease.

So, if you are a blood type A, and eat a great deal of meat, it will show up in the form of "indoles" or toxic substances through the Indican Scale urine test. He has repeatedly tested his patients and when they adhere to their blood type diets, the tests are benign, however, when they eat the offending foods for their blood types, the results will show up as indoles using the Indican Scale test.

Another interesting example of his findings are that blood type A's who consume foods with nitrites from bacon, ham, smoked foods or cold cuts, sustain far greater damage to their systems than a blood type O may sustain by eating the same food.

Chances are, if certain foods bother you, you will find those foods listed as foods to avoid in the D'Adamo diet. His findings may well be another piece to the puzzle of why certain people contract diseases more easily than others while living the same lifestyle.

We have to make some of our own health decisions and live with the results of those decisions, but it's easier if we have access to as much information as possible.

"Eat Right 4 (For) your Type" is a 391 page book and my minimal overview doesn't do his work justice.

EGGS—LUTEIN—YOUR EYES NEED "THOSE INCREDIBLE, EDIBLE EGGS."

I remember those catchy ads and how they disappeared after the "food scare" began, linking eggs, to cholesterol and heart disease. Millions of Americans were frightened to a point of "eggaphobia." Eggs were eliminated from diets, yet, heart disease continued to rise. Most recently the medical community has changed its hard-wired opposition to egg consumption and the American Medical Association has even suggested that multivitamins are a good idea.

Most probably because of a study conducted among 27,000 egg eaters and non-egg eaters. The study found that as a result of the elimination of eggs, important nutrients such as lutein, vitamin A, Vitamin B12, folate, vitamins E and C, were decreased among those non-egg eaters. (National Health and Nutritional Examination Survey (NHANES III, 1988-94). The results of the research appeared in the *Journal of the American College of Nutrition*—October 2000 (Supplement). Spinach, carrots, kale, and other leafy green vegetables are other good sources of lutein.

Multi-Vitamins, Lutein and macular degeneration

Researchers, Bill Sardi, and Dr. Stuart Richer, OD, PhD, (North Chicago Veterans Medical Center) have found that lutein also serves as a UV sun blocker for the retina. Their research, they believe, proves that macular degeneration is largely a deficiency disease and can be halted through, proper diet and supplementation with lutein. Their research was conducted for the Focus Foundation. "The Neural Retina: Lutein the Missing Carotenoid,"—"A 1980 study demonstrated that when lutein/zeaxanthin was removed from the diet of animals, signs of the retinal disease developed very rapidly (Inv Oph 1980; 19). It took until 1994 for a study, sponsored by Hoffman-LaRoche, to uncover the fact that individuals who consumed about 6 milligrams of lutein/zeaxanthin from spinach and other green leafy vegetables, experienced a significant decrease in the risk of macular degeneration (J Am Med Assoc 1994; 272). An ongoing NEI study of nutrients and retinal disease doesn't include lutein. Studies as early as 1948 showed lutein/zeaxanthin compounds improve visual adaptation to dim light and other studies published in 1956 and 1959 showed improvement among Retinitis Pigmentosa (RP) patients. Newborns are not born with this yellow spot. It has to be dietarily acquired (Retina 1981; 1) Hopefully the National Eye Institute will consider a clinical study of lutein/zeaxanthin given emerging evidence that it is involved in retinal degeneration."

They say "hopefully" when referring to the National Eye Institute conducting studies, however, that may be a long way off and there is adequate documentation presently available showing how a diet high in lutein protects vision. Again, lutein is found in eggs, spinach, carrots, yellow flowers (marigold), green leafy vegetables and kale.

In searching for the best formula for good eye health, it is important to make certain that your supplement contain 6 to 12 mg. of Lutein. Unfortunately, many respected name brands contain only 1/4 of one mg., not nearly enough, according to many alternative physicians. A good vitamin should also contain vitamin E, organic selenium (at least 50 mcg.), vitamin B12, magnesium, vitamin C, bilberry, DHA-rich fish oil—1000 mg of DHA; glutathione, lipoic acid, N-acetyl cysteine or taurine. Eating sulfur-rich foods, such as garlic, eggs, asparagus and onions are also helpful.

The good fats in our diet, such as olive oil and avocado, assist in transporting lutein to the retina. For what it's worth, among the many studies on lutein was an observation that smokers, blue-eyed persons and post-menopausal women have a more difficult time absorbing lutein. You may want to do more to be certain that you increase good absorption if you are in any of those groups. Of course, alternative physicians consider organic eggs the best.

FEVER CAN BE A BLESSING IN DISGUISE

For many years, the moment one of my children would show signs of a fever, I would rush for the Tylenol or aspirin bottle. That's what most people do when a cold or flu strikes. As parents, we don't want our children dealing with the discomfort of a fever. We behave as if fever were a disease and not a helpful process as well as a symptom. Only when we understand the medical mechanics of a fever, can we appreciate how our wondrously created bodies can be assisted by something as uncomfortable as a fever.

I received my education only after a visit to the emergency room with my oldest son who had been suffering classic flu symptoms with an accompanying fever. Our family doctor had been away. My first clue that the emergency room was not the place to be was in the fact that the doctor attending my son was sicker than my son! Not only did he have the flu but he, too, had a fever! My first thought was "What am I doing here?" I was quite anxious to get my wee one out of that emergency room. Dare I run for the door? I remained and went through the usual routine of being advised to give him fluid and rest.

The next day I advised our family doctor of what happened in his absence. He then sat me down and explained that fever is not a disease, but a symptom. He explained a fever is the body's way of defeating an invasion by bacteria and virus. He further explained that a moderate fever along with flu symptoms alone is not enough to warrant an emergency room visit. (I think he was attempting to advise me in gentle tones, that I was a little too overwrought as a parent). He even suggested that such hospital visits could expose us to other unnecessary risks and germs.

Germs proliferate at a temperature of around 98.6, according to our wise country doctor. When the body temperature rises, the fever kills off the offending germs. He suggested that I make certain to push fluids and hydrate my son and explained that the fever would keep my son still for a day or two while his body healed.

He then explained that when we take anti-fever medications, the body temperature drops to 98.6 and the germs go on to cheerfully reproduce because the anti-fever medications made it possible. I had never heard such a logical explanation. In reality, the doctor actually used high-powered medical terminology about endogenous pyrogens signaling the hypothalamus to raise the body temperature...metabolism increases, yada, yada, yada, but I preferred the English version.

Reducing fever should not be our first line of defense when attempting to comfort our children in cases of colds and flu, of course, unless the fever is exceptionally high. Fever also serves the purpose of keeping them quiet, allowing all of their energy to work on behalf of fighting the flu attack. Once the body temperature is back to normal because of medications, most children will bounce around and use their energy until the fever returns.

The common sense that was imparted to me made parenting a much more relaxed process. When we understand our body has such amazing built-in defense mechanisms, it is comforting.

He made it a point to explain that there are diseases and other conditions not related to the flu, where a fever should be of greater concern, especially high fevers or fevers that last for more than a few days.

One study suggested that cold remedies, Tylenol, and other preparations, might cause healing time from influenza to be prolonged. Researchers at the University of Maryland-Baltimore Schools of Pharmacy and Medicine conducted a vaccine study where volunteers were injected with various influenza vaccines, those volunteers administered drugs, suffered flu symptoms for an average 3.5 days longer than those who went entirely untreated. If taking aspirin or other anti-fever remedies reduce body temperature, then it stands to reason the flu germs would proliferate and "party" in one's system before they run their natural course.

Hopefully, my children will be better prepared than I was, at addressing some common illnesses without resorting to antibiotic therapy that has resulted in resistance among today's population.

FOLIC ACID: ESSENTIAL FOR MENTAL HEALTH AND GENERAL HEALTH

The nutrient is derived from the word "foliage," green, leafy vegetables. The nutrient is known as folate. It is more commonly called folacin or folic acid.

Very strangely, there have been blips on the television news programs here and there touting various small studies that show folic acid is not very useful. Now that's strange considering there is a large body of recognized evidence that proves that folic acid deficiencies result in birth defects, mental confusion and even depression. That leads me to question the protocols used in such studies. It's another of those nutrients that cannot be patented. In fact, sadly for the pharmaceuticals, it's a relatively inexpensive nutrient.

Jonathan Wright, M.D., another well-known alternative physician relates in his August 2004 newsletter that we should move folate to the top of our health priority list. He states that folate deficiency is extremely common in this nation. He then goes on to list five major health benefits of maintaining adequate levels of folate in the system. He explains that folate helps repair damaged DNA. Wright explains that damaged DNA can lead to various forms of cancer and that with adequate folate in the diet, the repairs of DNA can avert cancer-forming cells. He states in his August "Nutrition and Healing" newsletter, that "Colon cancer, rectal cancers, and adenomas—including benign, pre-cancerous and cancerous polyps—top the list of cancers preventable with adequate folate." He also points to other anti-cancer supplements such as vitamin D, selenium and iodine.

Science has already proven that folic acid reduces dangerous homocysteine levels, which is considered a major risk factor in developing heart disease. High homocysteine is also found in many patients with Alzheimer's disease. Wright states, "Adequate folate can help reduce your risk of Alzheimer's disease." Studies show that when combined with vitamin B6 and B12, a synergistic action takes place making folic acid even more effective.

Wright explains how adequate folates benefits human brain function and can help fight various forms of depression caused by folate deficiency. Folate deficiency, according to Wright, is one of the most common deficiencies we Americans suffer and perhaps could explain the ever-expanding use of anti-depressants in this country. Wright states, "Double-blind, placebo controlled studies have shown that the substance S-adenosylmethionine (SAM-e) has significant antidepressant effects. Folate is essential to our body's ability to make its own SAM-e."

On another front, from an article appearing on Dr. Joseph Mercola's web site, is a study that found folate to mitigate liver damage for those taking the drug Methotrexate, used for rheumatoid arthritis. Among patients in the study that appeared in the July 2001 issue of "Arthritis & Rheumatism," the incidence of toxicity from Methotrexate was greatly reduced among patients supplementing with folate. It was also noted that in some patients, the dosage of Methotrexate might have to be increased when supplementing with folate.

Now comes the problem. According to Wright, up to 50 percent of freshly available folate breaks down in green leafy vegetables within 48 hours of picking the vegetables. Additionally, we need adequate enzyme activity within our bodies to assimilate the folate properly. For that reason, I take "Folic Acid Hearts" which include B6 and B12. They cost about $5.00 for a 90 day supply—bad news for the pharmaceuticals.

Wright also states some of us may need much more than the minimum daily requirement and suggests all patients should obtain a test known as neutrophilic hypersegmentation index, which unfortunately most doctors don't require and many labs rarely offer. He explains the test will show how much folate your body is utilizing. For those who cannot find a place to obtain the test, he recommends having your physician draw the blood and send it to Meridian Valley Labs (425-271-8689). (www.meridianvalleylab.com).

There is a claim that one product can bypass the four-step conversion of folic acid by giving your body the exact form of folate it craves most and can immediately absorb—the active folate." The product name is HS Fighters and you can learn more about it or purchase it by calling 1-877-877-1970.

FLUORIDE—STUDY LINKS FLUORIDE TO GUM DISEASE

After watching a rerun of, "Dr. Strangelove," in which actor Sterling Hayden, portrays a paranoid, bomb-loving general, who decried that fluoridated water was sapping our (American) manhood, I've always been reticent to broach the topic, for fear of having someone remind me of the general's odd behavior.

The fact is, fluoride is a by-product of aluminum processing, known as silicofluoride, (not to be confused with natural occurring calcium fluoride). It was considered toxic in the early 1940's. I was a bit skeptical when I learned that Oscar Ewing, a lawyer for Alcoa Aluminum, headed the U.S. Public Health Service in the 1940's and began many experiments with fluoride.

I avoid fluoride whenever possible and most recently, I've discovered information that may boost my concerns about the substance.

So, what else is new? I ran across an astonishing article in the January 2003, issue of *Health Alert*, an alternative newsletter, regarding an application made by Sepracor Pharmaceutical for a patent to produce a drug to control "periodontal bone loss precipitated by fluoride." I checked the patent application on line and there it was. The application provides some interesting research.

The Sepracor application reads: "We have found that fluoride in the concentration range in which it is employed for the prevention of dental caries, (cavities) stimulates the production of prostaglandins and thereby exacerbates the inflammatory response in gingivitis and periodontitis—thus the including of fluoride in toothpastes and mouthwashes for the purpose of inhibiting the development of caries (cavities) may, at the same time, accelerate the process of chronic destructive periodontitis."

This is news! The answer by Sebracor is to produce a fluoride/anti-inflammatory combination drug, which should be addressed in a separate article.

Once you learn that a product or additive is an inflammatory agent, wouldn't logic tell you that the risks outweigh the benefits?

So, if the pharmaceutical has determined through their research that fluoride is causing inflammation and contributing to the break down of gums and dental bone, what is it doing to the rest of our body when we ingest it?

The latest medical research available points to the inflammation process as being associated with heart disease and many other diseases across the board. The latest pharmaceutical research has found that fluoride creates inflammation! Other recent research also shows an association between the toxic metal, aluminum and Alzheimer's. Pardon the high-powered language, but "helloooo!" Doesn't it seem that scientists should get together on this? Inflammation seems to be the common thread in the disease process.

If the Sebracor research is correct, shouldn't periodontists be advised? Shouldn't dentists be telling patients with gingivitis to stop using toothpastes and products containing fluoride?

After all, in a March, 1984 editorial in *The Journal of the American Dental Association*, it was pointed out that 84% of dental caries among 5 to 17 year-olds involved tooth surfaces with pits and fissures where fluorides could not be expected to reach and protect. The article advised sealants were effective for these areas. If 84% of cavities (among 5 to 17 year-olds) cannot be addressed by fluoride because of cavity location, doesn't risk vs. benefits come into even greater play?

There are a number of countries that have eliminated or are in the process of eliminating fluoridation, based on their own studies. Belgium is even considering a ban on fluoride in toothpaste. According to *Health Alert* publishers, "because their own Health Ministry found that excessive use of fluoride products could cause fluoride poisoning, damage to the central nervous system and osteoporosis." (Reuter's 07/13/02)

There is a great deal of research out there and only one of the numerous footnotes from the fluoridedebate.com site explains "Dr. John Colquhoun, Principal Dental Officer, in Auckland, New Zealand's largest city, wrote "…tooth decay had declined, but there was virtually no difference in tooth decay rates between the fluoridated and non-fluoridated places. Those (statistics) for 1981 showed that in most Health Districts the percentage of 12-and 13-year-old children who were free of tooth decay—that is, had perfect teeth—was greater in the non fluoridated part of the district." (See 1-10: "Why I Changed My Mind About Water Fluoridation," *Perspectives in Biology and Medicine*. 41,1 autumn 1997, University of Chicago

It seems that all roads lead to good nutrition. A healthy diet, less sugar and proper dental hygiene are the best roads to both dental and general health.

GASTRIC REFLUX—GERD

Many conventional physicians treat symptoms rather than causes of disorders Americans especially, tend to want the "quick fix" and become impatient with the time and effort involved in correcting many complaints. One such disorder for which millions of Americans take antacids or prescription medications, is a condition known as gastroesophageal reflux disease (GERD) or "reflux." It is estimated that as many as forty percent of Americans, including little ole me, on occasion, have at least a small degree of esophageal reflux. Twenty percent have persistent and weekly episodes of what is referred to as "heartburn."

The condition occurs when stomach acids go in an upward backflow. Persistent heartburn can create serious problems. The esophagus is unable to protect itself with any type of lining and the backflow of acids and other stomach contents can cause disorders that can eventually lead to cancer.

According to the authors of *Disease Prevention and Treatment,* "The condition is aggravated in persons who are smokers, overweight, or pregnant. A person who eats fried, fatty or spicy food; eats chocolate, peppermint and citrus fruits, or drinks coffee, tea, alcohol and carbonated drinks can also experience reflux because these substances can increase the tendency of the esophageal sphincter to relax." It is suggested that patients avoid eating for at least three hours prior to going to bed and that they eat small amounts of food at more frequent intervals, rather than 3 large meals. This practice has mostly eliminated my problem.

The authors warn that many people who take certain medications for GERD may not attempt to change lifestyle and eating habits once the medications resolve their pain. That is dangerous, they explain, because histamine 2 (H2) receptor antagonist drugs, such as "Tagamet, Pepcid, Zantac and Axid relieve symptoms, "they do not prevent damage done to the esophagus by acid, enzymes, bile, and other stomach contents."

Another class of GERD medications known as proton-pump inhibitors, such as Nexium, Prilosec and Prevacid, can heal most all of the esophagitis cases, but according to the authors, can also create problems when used long-term. "There is a theory that these acid-suppressing drugs will reduce esophageal cancer risk by preventing acid irritation. Evidence, however, shows that long-term use of proton-pump suppressing drugs may not only increase esophageal cancer risk, but other digestive tract cancers as well," state the authors. They clarify that the above drugs create such a low stomach acid that the stomach pushes to secrete a hormone called "gastrin" in an attempt to further produce stomach acid. Excess levels of gastrin, the authors write: "are associated with a host of digestive tract cancers." They further point out that over the last 25 years, esophageal cancer has increased by 350%.

Thankfully, the authors point to various studies including a Yale University study that found that people who ate fresh vegetables, beta-carotene, folate, vitamins C, B6 and fiber had a lower risk of cancers of the esophagus and stomach.

Alternative physicians believe the entire gastrointestinal system must be placed into balance and that something as simple as replacing the friendly bacteria in the intestines by adding various forms of acidophilus to the diet, will begin to create that balance. They test for food allergies, which they feel, can trigger reflux and recommend enzyme products that will help us better digest our foods. In fact, Dr. Joseph Mercola of Schaumburg, Il. states that GERD is one of the disorders that he has treated with great success. His first suggestion is to add acidophilus to the diet.

We tend to take medications rather than address the causes and take necessary measures to eliminate the condition.

Reflux can cause us to avoid eating our vegetables. We all need our phyto-chemicals (plant foods-vegetables) and if we cannot digest them properly, we lose the necessary benefits they provide in nourishing and protecting our bodies from disease.

The bottom line is that we need stomach acid to digest our foods and relieving the symptoms of indigestion is not enough. The cause of indigestion must be found and treated. The human body was created to produce acid and enzymes to assist us in breaking down our foods in order to utilize the vitamins and other nutrients that help us survive.

For those who do not eat their vegetables, there is a newer phyto-chemical multi-vitamin available from Great American Products. Keeping in mind that nothing is as good as the "real McCoy" when seeking nutrient benefits; the new multi-vitamin includes phyto-chemicals as well as components of green tea. "Green Supreme Multi Vitamin" from Great American Products, can be purchased at: 800-242-1223. Additionally, Life Extension Foundation recommends digestive aids. You can inquire at 800-544-4440 or go to www.lef.org. Your local health food store will also carry digestive aids as well as phyto-nutrients.

GOUT: CONVENTIONAL AND ALTERNATIVE TREATMENTS

Gout is a very painful arthritic disorder that affects approximately 840 out of every 100,000 Americans, mostly men between the ages of 40 to 50. I decided to visit the Arthritis Foundation web site and other conventional web sites around the world to gather as much information as possible about gout. I then searched for the conventional treatments after which I performed yet another search for information on how gout is treated in the alternative community and what alternative physicians had to say about cause and treatment.

What is gout?

Gout is a form of arthritis. It was said to be the disease of kings because it was seen among those who ate the richest of foods. Gout can cause severe pain in only one or two joints with each attack. The ball of the big toe is one of the most common affected joints. The skin over the joint may become red, shiny and swollen.

What causes Gout?

Gout occurs when there is too much uric acid in the blood. Uric acid results from the breakdown of purines, which are part of all human tissue and are found in many foods. Generally, uric acid is dissolved in the blood and is processed through the kidneys then eliminated through urination. When our body fails to eliminate the uric acid, and higher levels build up in the blood, the uric acid crystals can accumulate in the joint spaces causing inflammation. The crystals can also collect in the kidney causing kidney stones. Uric acid is a chemical in the blood, needed to break down food, but when it is over-produced and not dissolved properly, gout may occur. High alcohol intake, especially beer and wine, can raise uric acid levels; some blood pressure medications (diuretics) can also result in increased uric acid blood levels. Because of the problems with processing purine, it is recommended that high purine diets be avoided. People with gout also may have an enzyme defect that interferes with the body's ability to process high purine foods. High purine diets, include liver, kidneys, tripe, shellfish, peas, lentils, and beans. All of these high-purine foods have a tendency to irritate the condition and bring on attacks. Obesity is another culprit, but we should all realize by now that obesity can contribute to almost any disease.

An interesting observation is found in the *Journal of the American Medical Association*, May 10, 2000, in which they discuss a 16 year study that found a nexus among those with consistently high uric acid levels and heart disease which may well confirm the alternative medicine theory that all disease is inter-related and the cause of one disease may well be the cause of many. Conversely, they believe that foods that fight one disease will fight many diseases.

Conventional therapy:

Conventional therapies very wisely advise dietary changes, which include remaining on a low purine diet, weight loss when necessary and prescription medications to control the pain. Water intake should be increased, especially when taking medications for gout, to help alleviate the possibility of forming kidney stones. Commonly used prescription medications include, Allopurinol, which inhibits uric acid synthesis, Colchicine, Probenecid and Indomethacin a non-steroidal anti-inflammatory drug (NSAID). I checked the Physicians Desk Reference pertaining to all of the drugs used for gout, and each of them of them were shown to have possible toxic side effects. NSAID's have become the treatment of choice among physicians, and while they can also produce toxic side-effects, they are generally less dangerous if used only for short term purposes.

Alternative therapy

The basis of alternative therapy is that most all disease has some basic nexus and that treating symptoms is merely masking the basic cause of disease. Alternative physicians believe that the digestive system is ultimately the core of many diseases and if the food we eat is not processed properly, we will begin to display many disorders that are believed to be signs of deficiencies in either diet or the digestion process.

The alternative remedies I have located suggest the same basic dietary prohibitions as the conventional community, however, alternative physicians believe that digestive enzymes should be part of the treatment. They also feel that milk and some other dairy products are culprits and should be avoided. Foods that are recommended to help fight gout are brown rice, cherries, strawberry, oranges, dates, fresh coconut, avocados, honey raisins, only sour dairy products, chestnuts, uncooked almonds, bananas, apples, pears, strawberries, oranges, celery and celery seed, carrots, unsweetened juices (no cranberry). Note: According to Dr. Susan Lark, celery seed contains 25 anti-inflammatory agents.

The recommended supplements to the diet are anti-inflammatories such as bromelain, quercetin, turmeric, garlic, silymarin, black cherry, celery seed and potassium citrate. There are two companies that combine these ingredients and you may wish to seek further information on the products. One company that combines the above ingredients is Young Again at 1-877-205-0040. Remember, when supplementing with anything, always consult with your physician first.

HEART DISEASE: CAUSES AND TREATMENT—CAN HEART DISEASE BE ASSOCIATED WITH LEAD IN THE SYSTEM?

Could it be that some cases of heart disease are actually caused by lead poisoning? That's exactly what Dr. Robert Jay Rowen believes. Rowen writes in the October 2003, issue of his "Second Opinion" newsletter that prior to the 1980s, accepted safe numbers for blood levels of lead have been drastically reduced due to more recent research showing the dangers of even small amounts of lead in the blood. He points to the mid 1960s, when a diagnosis of lead poisoning was determined if blood levels were above 60 mcg. per deciliter (mcg/dl). That is a level high enough to cause kidney and brain damage as well as abdominal spasms. However, in the 1980s and 1990s, the Centers for Disease Control and Prevention (CDC) reduced the danger level to 25 mcg. Again, in 1991 it was reduced to 10 mcg. Even at 10 mcg. lead has been shown to create health problems including mental decline and sexual dysfunction.

Rowen states we are now learning that lead poisoning actually occurs at a fraction of presently accepted levels and could be the cause of many health problems including heart disease. He cites a study conducted at the University of Maryland in which researchers followed 2,165 women aged 40-59 years. The study, according to Rowen, found that even low levels of lead exposure appeared to have a correlation to hypertension. Low lead levels were found to have interrupted electrical rhythm and elasticity of the vascular smooth muscle tissue as well as having adverse affects on renal control mechanisms of blood pressure.

Rowen believes even low levels of lead contamination can create ill effects throughout the system. He further refers to a recent study published in the *New England Journal of Medicine* (NEJM) that indicated IQ levels of children fell by 4.6 points for every 10 mcg. rise in lead levels above 10 mcg. The article in NEJM quotes the researchers as concluding, "Blood lead concentrations, even those below 10 mcg per deciliter, are inversely associated with children's IQ scores at three and five years of age, and associated declines in IQ are greater at these concentrations than at higher concentrations. These findings suggest that more U.S. children may be adversely affected by environmental lead than previously estimated." The studies among children have implications for those of us who were tested many years ago and found to have "safe" levels of lead at any measure under 60 mcg. These are levels that are now considered extremely dangerous.

Candles, paint, gasoline, dishes, air, toys as a lead source

We assume we are much safer today because laws were enacted to discontinue use of lead in paints, gasoline and certain plastic products. Not exactly true. A source of lead I just learned of is found in some candle wicks. I find candle burning to be calming, and relaxing; however, recently I learned that lead had been used to stiffen some candlewicks and unfortunately, even though the law is designed to include the wicks, some still contain lead. Part of the problem lies in the fact that many of our candles are imported, especially from China. Other countries do not have the rigid safety parameters that the United States regulatory agencies require for American companies. You may remember that recently, painted toys from China were found to contain lead paint. Only small percentages of goods imported into the U.S. are examined at all. The high standards basically apply to American manufacturers, not to those importing to the U.S. It makes me wonder if some of those foggy headed politicians haven't sucked on a few too many paint chips as children. But that's another story.

Additionally, the Environmental Protection Agency states that homes built prior to 1978—possibly 75 percent of those homes—may have a far greater chance of containing lead paint or other lead-containing building materials and pipe solder that have since been banned. Even fluoride in our water supply has been shown to cause both lead and aluminum absorption.

If you feel you have been exposed to lead, you might be wise to suggest your doctor obtain your blood lead levels. For testing water and various other surfaces, you can purchase lead testing kits by calling Professional Equipment 800-334-9291, Abotex water test 888-438-1942, or pick up lead testing kits at Kroger, Whole Foods, or GNC Vitamins. You can also inquire at your local hardware store.

Heart disease detected through your breath

Sometimes, it takes modern science awhile to latch onto a concept that is so obviously plausible and workable. I know it doesn't sound too appealing, but for many years, doctors would observe a patient's breath to get an indication of underlying disease. Various breath odors are very good indicators of disorders. For instance, when a person has diabetes, his/her breath will smell sweet and fruity. If the breath has an ammonia or urine-like odor, kidney disease is the likely culprit. In serious liver disease, doctors notice a musty fishy odor. A fresh bread smell might indicate typhoid fever and foul breath along with other symptoms of fatigue may indicate mononucleosis.

Most of us are aware of the use of the Breathalyzer for detecting inebriated drivers. The Breathalyzer measures alcohol. It can measure with pretty good accuracy the amount of alcohol that the driver has consumed.

There is a new machine similar to the Breathalyzer that does basically the same thing to determine the presence of various diseases. It is a billion times more sensitive than the Breathalyzer and measures volatile organic compounds (VOC's) to determine what diseases may be present. The machine has already been proven to determine early signs of heart transplant rejection before symptoms materialize. The new Heartsbreath machine by Mensanna Research, Inc., has been approved for heart transplant patients; however, it is showing tremendous value for detecting other diseases in ongoing clinical trials. The ultra-sensitive machine is capable of detecting over 200 chemicals that help diagnose various conditions from cancer to organ rejection. The promise of the new machine is that it will detect disorders early on when they can be more successfully treated. Another major advantage of the new breath machine is that it will also help patients avoid uncomfortable biopsies. The Food & Drug Administration (FDA) has already approved similar machines that help in the detection of asthma and stomach ulcers. Presently, there are clinical trials being conducted to study the markers that show up in heart disease, diabetes, lung cancer and even schizophrenia. The machine is being tested with funding from the National Institutes of Health to hasten its move to the marketplace for detecting these other diseases. In one early trial, it has already been shown to detect 80 percent of early lung cancers.

Every year in the United States, 99,000 men and 78,000 women develop lung cancer. Dr. Michael Phillips, the developer of the machine, believes that if the lung cancer is localized at the time of diagnosis and treated promptly, the five-year survival rate will be tripled. Such an early screening test will have the potential to reduce the lung cancer death rate appreciably.

Physicians using the machine merely ask the patient to sit quietly for several minutes while breathing into a steel cigarette-like tube. The tube is then capped and each gas and chemical is measured. It is so sensitive, that it is necessary to also measure the air components in the room air in which the test is being taken. Certain compounds show up as indicating the presence of various diseases. This machine is almost like something Dr. McCoy might have used in his Star Trek adventures.

I suspect this non-invasive procedure will move forward quickly, especially since some of the early results of clinical trials have shown it to be as effective as suggested.

I will follow the progress of these studies closely and will report any new information as soon as it becomes available. I hope to obtain a list of physicians and medical centers using this new equipment. It's always a step forward to be able to eliminate uncomfortable biopsies whenever possible.

HEART TEST: YOU CAN DO IT AT HOME

When physicians write prescriptions for numerous diagnostic procedures and blood tests, they are hoping to either confirm or rule out various conditions. The fact is, the tests are usually very expensive and money will always be a major consideration to the patient in determining which tests he or she will actually obtain. When we consider deductibles, co-pays or even self-pay, the idea of many of these expensive tests is a joke.

For the above reasons I was very interested in a number of simple tests used to determine heart risks by some alternative physicians. The tests can be conducted at home (for the most part) without any equipment other than a tape measure, a watch and two fingers. The first test involves recording pulse rates during and shortly after exercise. It is known as a "Cardiac Recovery Test," and has been written of by medical researcher and biochemist, Bruce West as well as Brian Vont, M.D. and Joseph Mercola, D.O. Dr. Vont also lists various other simple at-home tests that can be taken to help determine general heart health. They believe the tests will establish if you are at risk for heart attack or stroke at the present time.

Test number one is performed by exercising to around peak or 85 percent of peak heart output levels (220 minus your age) on a treadmill, Stairmaster or when performing regular exercise. During peak exercise you should record your pulse, according to the doctors. You must again take your pulse one minute after stopping exercise. After one minute, "Your pulse should drop by 20 to 30 beats. If not, your heart is not in good shape" according to West. West goes so far as to state, "if it drops less than 12 beats, you are at a higher risk for a heart attack."

Of course, it should be understood that patients already diagnosed with heart disease or extremely obese people, as well as those who do not exercise regularly, should not perform the test unless monitored in a medical facility.

Another helpful indicator, according to the doctors, is in merely recording your resting heart rate. This is basically a test for men because in women this particular test does not show the same correlation with women. Dr. Mercola believes that a highly elevated resting heart rate is an indicator of possible cardiovascular disease in men.

A healthy resting rate is described as being below 64 beats/min. Very few people I know of run at that rate. They consider a mild risk to be between 64 to 69 beats per minute. Moderate risk is believed to be 70 to 75 beats per minute, while high risk is between 76 to 80 beats per minute. Above 80 beats per minute, according to Dr. Mercola, the risk is much higher.

Another factor in Dr. Vont's article is the suggestion that patient's measure their waist size as well as height. If your waist size in inches is greater than one-half of your height in inches, he believes it adds to your relative risk factors. The greater your abdominal girth relative to your height, the greater your chances of cardiovascular disease, according to Dr. Vont. He also mentions that actuarial tables used by insurance companies, involve measuring your height, weight and waist size for the very reason of determining these risks.

Naturally, blood work and other diagnostic measures when used along with these tests, will give the most accurate assessment of your general heart health, but these tests can give a bird's eye view of your general condition according to West, Vont and Mercola. Mercola's web site www.mercola.com also lists several additional measures that can be taken to check other factors that may be involved in creating heart difficulties. Use the key word "heart rate recovery" to locate the Vont article.

It's important to realize that even if these scores are not what we would want, we can change our diet and add exercise to assure better health. An even better bonus is in realizing that a better diet along with exercise will prove helpful in boosting the entire system, not just the heart.

HEMOCHROMATOSIS OR HEPATITIS C?

It wasn't until I began reading background on Hepatitis C that I learned of hepatitis C being misdiagnosed or even caused by a condition known as hemochromatosis (iron overload). The symptoms are pretty much the same. Hemochromatosis is the most common inherited disease afflicting people of Eastern European descent. It is also an often overlooked disease.

Dr. Joseph Mercola wrote of his experience with the case of a 53-year old patient who had been diagnosed with Hepatitis C. The man was healthy and through his regular check-up and routine blood tests, it was discovered he had elevated liver enzymes. A hepatitis panel was drawn and the patient was confirmed to have hepatitis C. The patient was then referred for treatment with interferon, the protocol conventional physicians use to treat the disease. The man had read of the possibility of hemochromatosis among patients diagnosed with Hepatitis C and refused to accept his diagnosis without further consultation. He also refused to accept the 30 percent "cure" rate of interferon, so he decided to see Dr. Mercola for a second opinion.

At the patient's insistence, his original physician ordered a serum iron test. It came back high/normal, and the doctors concluded their original diagnosis of hepatitis C was correct. According to Dr. Mercola, there is a more intricate series of blood tests needed to make a conclusive determination of hemochromatosis. The most important issue to Dr. Mercola was that this patient was fortunate to have refused the interferon treatment that would have actually caused him harm.

When Mercola drew the man's ferritin blood levels they were at an astonishing 1000. A good number is 50, according to Mercola. He writes, "The most useful laboratory test to ascertain hemochromatosis is measuring serum iron concentration, total iron binding capacity, transferrin saturation and serum ferritin. These should be done together." In some cases a diagnosis of Hepatitis C is made without these additional tests to rule out hemochromatosis, which is treated differently than Hepatitis C.

Mercola points out that 15 percent of the world's population has an iron deficiency, however, 20 percent of Americans have iron overload. Americans who eat meat three or four times per week or take supplements with iron, can have difficulty in excreting the excess iron stores.

Conventional Vs. Alternative treatment of hemochromatosis

Once the additional tests are conducted to determine a diagnosis of hemochromatosis, the conventional treatment consists of drawing blood on a regular basis to reduce the blood iron levels. According to Dr. Mercola, this is an "inelegant" and time-consuming practice. Mercola states he reduces iron levels by using iron-based chelators such as phytic acid (IP6), which is derived from rice bran and is relatively inexpensive. It binds to iron and helps remove excess iron from the system, according to Mercola. There is no regular drawing of blood except for testing purposes. Phytic acid (IP6) only became commercially available in 1998.

What is good for the liver?

The authors of Health Science Institute newsletter state, N-acetylcysteine (NAC) stimulates production of glutathione, a most potent antioxidant enzyme. "This ability to infuse the liver with antioxidants, coupled with excellent anti-inflammatory properties, makes NAC an effective liver crisis treatment. Studies have shown that NAC treatments may significantly decrease the chance of mortality in patients suffering from acute liver damage," claim the authors of Health Science Institute.

The authors additionally report that milk thistle (silymarin) has been shown to stimulate the production of new liver cells, and helps protect the liver from alcohol damage. It is also used to treat liver diseases. The publication also reports, "Turmeric root, like NAC, is reputed to have powerful antioxidant and anti-inflammatory effects that promote healthy liver function. And burdock helps to stimulate the liver's ability to purify the blood." Vitamins C and E are also good antioxidants for the liver as well as B-vitamins, zinc and lecithin., alpha lipoic acid, selenium, NAC, and herbs such as milk thistle and burdock are all written of by alternative physician as helpful for the liver.

Many years ago, an old country doctor ordered my mom to squeeze 1/2 a lemon into 8 ounces of warm water on a daily basis. He told her it would help her cleanse her liver. We laughed at his comment that "lemon is the liver's friend." It seemed so silly. Now, as I read various articles on liver health from alternative sources, freshly squeezed lemon juice is always a component of any liver cleansing program. Dr. Sinatra supports fresh lemon juice as part of his liver health program. He states the fresh squeezed juice assists liver metabolism. Additionally, Sinatra suggests that foods like artichokes have potent bioflavonoid activity, which has positive effects on stimulating bile.

Sinatra even suggests supplementing with artichoke in pill form. Then there is natural cranberry juice. He recommends mixing crushed flaxseed or psyllium seed with a glass of natural cranberry juice in 8 oz. of water and drinking it as a liver flush. (No cranberry juice for those with gout). Milk thistle (silymarin) is another major aspect of Dr. Sinatra's healthy liver program. Sinatra says, "Milk thistle not only blocks the effects of multiple liver toxins, but also helps regenerate damaged liver cells, nurturing them back to full efficiency." Other vital nutrients in his liver program include the amino acid, L-carnitine that he says, "helps detoxify lactic acidosis and ammonia, both of which are extraordinarily toxic to the liver." He further explains, "L-carnitine protects the liver from metabolic breakdown of alcohol as well."

As always, Sinatra's major concern is that his patients adopt a Pan Asian Modified Mediterranean (PAMM) diet. This includes more fresh vegetables, fish, and extra virgin olive oil instead of butters or margarine. Under the chapter on "Hepatitis C" I wrote of Dr. Burt Berkson's use of alpha lipoic acid for liver assistance. I also covered the role of N-Acetyl cysteine (NAC) in treating liver poisoning from overdosing on acetaminophen.

Our intake of excess sugar, alcohol, heavy metals, insecticides, statin drugs for cholesterol, Tylenol (acetaminophen), caffeine, and many other products stress the liver, causing impaired liver function. He also warns about taking high dose vitamin A (retinol palmitate), of over 15,000 IU's because the liver has difficulty in eliminating the high-dose fats. He says taking under 7,500 IU's of beta-carotene is okay.

Understanding the function of your liver

Many of us have little understanding of the tremendous role healthy liver function plays in keeping us alive and well—and thin. We also know little about the daily assaults our liver suffers from environmental factors as well as from prescribed and over-the counter medicines.

The liver is an organ located on the right side of the body, just under the rib cage. It acts as a filter to cleanse our blood. It helps us absorb vitamins and good fats, aids in digestion, assist with production of hormones, manufactures cholesterol (too much if it's not healthy) and even help the body eliminate bacteria. Those are just a few of the many functions of an organ we rarely think about. But then, pondering our liver function might make us really weird, boring people.

HEPATITIS B VACCINE—ARE YOU REALLY AT HIGH RISK?

How would you feel if you knew that the latest universally recommended immunization program for infants and children included a shot, formerly used only for children of IV drug users, prostitutes and other promiscuous or high-risk types?

How would you feel if you knew that that shot for hepatitis-B resulted in more serious reactions than cases of the disease itself? How would you feel if your son and daughter-in-law's beautiful triplet boys who were several days away from being released from the hospital, instead ended up in the neonatal intensive care unit; the smallest doing very poorly, possibly in part, because of a hepatitis-B shot?

"Meningitis" my son told me. "They think it's meningitis?"

In shock, I asked what happened and my son informed me that the boys had been given their hepatitis-B shot and began showing signs of everything from lethargy with the smallest one so unresponsive, he seemed paralyzed. They were all very pale in color. The little guy was diagnosed with possible meningitis, but after puncturing his tiny spine, they determined it wasn't meningitis. Blood work showed he had group-B strep, a dangerous infection, with no one willing to explain the cause.

Of course, the relationship to the hepatitis-B shot may have been questioned in one baby of three; but, another unrelated baby who was also prepared to go home was now back in ICU as well. The problem with the other premature baby also began with the immunization. Another coincidence I suppose. Considering premature babies are already struggling to reach parity with full-term babies, why would anyone do something so illogical as give that particular shot?

What immediately rang a bell with me was yet another "coincidence" wherein my great niece was also rushed to the emergency room, diagnosed with possible meningitis after getting her hepatitis-B shot. Coincidence seems to abound.

When I got the news, my first reaction was to contact church-going friends and family to ask for a prayer chain for the boys. I then went to work throughout that night and the next few days, gathering information on hepatitis-B and the hepatitis-B immunization.

I found several web sites related to vaccines and I was especially interested in the credentials of Dr. Burton Waisbren, author of *The Hepatitis-B Vaccination Program in the United States—Lessons for the Future.* He began his research in 1976 on reactions to the swine flu vaccination and found many similarities to hepatitis-B reactions.

I had been up all night and it was now 8:00 a.m., so I sent a short e-mail to Dr. Waisbren explaining the circumstances—praying he would somehow read this desperate plea from a total stranger.

Five minutes later—my phone rang and on the other end of the line was the kind voice of Dr. Burton Waisbren! In my entire lifetime, I have never had my own doctor return a call so quickly! I was blown away. Dr. Waisbren, wanted to know the immediate conditions of the babies and offered his services to the triplets' pediatrician, should it have been a reaction to the hepatitis-B shot. He explained he knew of several helpful procedures in certain cases of hepatitis-B reaction. He also explained the shot was responsible for many reactions, and that he was aware of another case exactly as that of our triplets. We all thank God that within 4 days the babies were improved, however, they remained in the neonatal ICU for observation.

In my quest for information, I learned that in France, all school age hepatitis B immunizations were suspended in 1998. There were questions of an increase in autoimmune diseases such as rheumatoid arthritis among school-age children who received the hepatitis-B shot. They continue to allow infant immunization.

I have learned that there are a great number of physicians who are opposed to hepatitis-B immunization entirely, except in cases of high-risk parents and children. I also learned that there have been over 24,100, reactions to the hepatitis-B shot from 1990 to 1998, with one-third resulting in hospitalization and many resulting in death. Reactions are most likely under-reported since independent studies found that approximately only 10% to 18% of American doctors file such reports. It is necessary to fill out a "Vaccination Adverse Event Report" (VAERS) and many doctors just don't take the time.

Dr. Joseph Mercola writes, "Hepatitis B is a rare, mainly blood-transmitted disease. In 1996 only 54 cases of the disease were reported to the CDC in the 0-1 age group. There were 3.9 million births that year, so the observed incidence of hepatitis B in the 0-1 age group was just 0.001%. In the Vaccine Adverse Event Reporting System (VAERS), there were 1,080 total reports of adverse reactions from hepatitis B vaccine in 1996 in the 0-1 age group, with 47 deaths reported."

So what should parents know about the hepatitis B vaccine?

On October 8, 1998, the Associated Press headline read:

"French Suspend Hepatitis B Inoculations,—Faced with a potential health disaster, France has suspended hepatitis B vaccine inoculations of school children 4 years after the mass immunization program began."

The reason? Too many reactions including autoimmune symptoms. In 2001, French neuro-pathologist, Romain Gherardi, made a discovery while investigating macrophagic myofasciitis (MMF), which appears to be somewhat like chronic fatigue syndrome. The disorder was reported in 1998. Gherardi noted aluminum hydroxide, a component of the hepatitis B, hepatitis A and tetanus immunizations, appeared in the muscle tissue of many patients tested for the disease. Dr. Gherardi, believes the epidemiological survey, now being conducted in France, may substantiate the possible link between aluminum hydroxide in vaccines, and some of the autoimmune diseases being reported. He feels it may also provide insight into what is known as Gulf War Syndrome.

In his book, *The Hepatitis B vaccination program in the United States—Lessons for the future*, Burton Waisbren, M.D., explains that two of the scientists involved in the development of the hepatitis B vaccine, Dr. M.R. Hilleman and Dr. Arie Zuckerman, both initally expressed concerns about the vaccine as early as 1975, one, even suggesting that a vaccine against the disease, might create problems with autoimmunity.

Dr. Weisberg noted during the swine flu immunization program in the 1970's, that many of those having severe adverse reactions to the vaccine were displaying autoimmune symptoms. The more recently reported hepatitis B immunizations were once again, drawing his attention because of the reactions.

The more serious adverse events included Guillain-Barre Syndrome, multiple sclerosis, postvaccinal encephalomyelitis, optic neuritis, meningoencephalitis and other demyelinating diseases.

Trust the experts?

Keep in mind the fact that most of "the experts" have refused to take the smallpox vaccine. There are estimated to be over 100,000 deaths in the U.S. each year, attributable to adverse drug reactions and approximately 1.5 million hospitalizations from drug reactions. A rotavirus immunization for infants, approved by "experts" resulted in the deaths of 14 infants with many others requiring surgery for bowel obstructions after immunization. The rotavirus vaccine was voluntarily withdrawn from the list of available vaccines in 1999, only 18 months after it was approved.

Remember the Thalidomide tragedy, Fen-phen, and Rezulin? Vioxx? Baycol? FDA approved drugs are often being removed from the market quickly after being approved. How did they become approved in the first place? "Experts" approved them.

Then consider that the Illinois Dept. of Public Health website states that hepatitis B is not easily spread; certainly not through casual contact. The website further states: "Most patients with mild to severe hepatitis B, begin to feel better in two to three weeks and have complete recovery in four to eight weeks." Does this justify mass inoculation of every child not at risk, even considering the adverse reactions? The U.S. has reached a point where we are having more reactions than cases of the disease. Even worse, the CDC admits the new 5 in 1 shots containing the hepatitis B virus, will probably result in even more reactions.

Question of a link between Hepatitis B vaccine and MS

A September 16, 2004 news report prepared by the British Broadcasting Corporation (BBC) disclosed that studies conducted in the United States concluded, "People who are vaccinated against hepatitis B are at an increased risk of developing multiple sclerosis (MS), according to a study of UK patients." It further disclosed, "American public health experts discovered a link between the vaccine and MS when they examined records of more than 1,500 people. The research team does not know if the vaccine causes MS of those already susceptible to the disease or if it speeds up the onset."

An interesting observation is that in the 1990's there were concerns among some researchers in the U.S. that the Hepatitis B vaccine might have a correlation to MS, however, studies at that time, disputed the claim. Since that time, at least some of the original researchers have changed their minds because additional study patients have developed MS. There is no suggestion that the hepatitis B vaccine is what causes all cases of MS. In fact approximately 90% of the people afflicted with MS have not had the Hepatitis B vaccine. However, there may well be a link between hepatitis B vaccination and the other 10% of MS cases.

The BBC report also explained that "In the latest study Dr Miguel Hernan and colleagues looked at people registered with a GP in the United Kingdom who had been diagnosed with MS between 1993 and 2000. When they looked at hepatitis B immunization patterns among these 163 MS patients and 1,604 'control' patients without MS from the same GP database, they found a link between the vaccine and MS. Dr Hernan said: "We estimated that immunisation against hepatitis B was associated with a three-fold increase in the incidence of MS within three years following vaccination."

Let's look at "risk versus benefits." About 50 percent of patients who contract Hepatitis B will have no symptoms but will have lifetime immunity to the disease. About 30 percent will develop flu-like symptoms and there have been reports of 25,000 reactions from 1990 to 1998. These include deaths. Keep in mind that most adverse reactions are not even reported by doctors. So the figure of 25,000 reactions from 1990 to 1998 most likely is far higher.

Dr. Mercola goes on to say, "Let us put this in simpler terms. For every child with hepatitis B there were 20 that were reported to have severe complications. Let us also remember that only 10% of the reactions are reported to VAERS, so this means: Traditional medicine is harming 200 children to protect one from hepatitis B."

It is important to also keep in mind that two of the disputing studies were partially funded by the manufacturers of the vaccines.

Always, follow the money. In the meantime, learn how to build a healthy immune system naturally.

MEDICAL CONFLICTS OF INTEREST WITH HEPATITIS B VACCINE APPROVAL?

Two Center for Disease Control (CDC) employees who promoted the universal hepatitis B immunization were Dr. Harold Margolis and David West, Ph.D. Dr. Burton Waisbren writes: "Dr. West resigned from the CDC and went to work for Merck and Company, the main manufacturer of hepatitis B vaccine. Shortly after the program was announced, he wrote articles in medical journals supporting the (hepatitis B) experiment. Dr. Margolis appointed a vaccine advisory committee made up of academians and industry. The majority of the academians were receiving grants from the government." Merck earns about one billion a year from the hepatitis B vaccine.

The Illinois Senate passed a simple "conflict of interest" law. The bill merely required that all members of the vaccine advisory committee have no financial interest or ties to pharmaceutical manufacturers. Governor Ryan vetoed the bill. His reason for the veto was that it is almost impossible to eliminate conflicts of interest. Nonsense, there are many good doctors who have no ties to pharmaceuticals and they should be considered for appointment to the vaccine advisory committee.

What can be done?

Most physicians who are concerned about the hepatitis B immunization state that pregnant mothers should be tested for hepatitis B and if they are positive, only their children should be vaccinated.

Contact your legislators if you believe this shot should not be mandatory or given to all infants at birth. Only when parents demand action, will legislators act with responsibility. It's about your children.

HEPATITIS C—CONVENTIONAL AND ALTERNATIVE TREATMENTS

There are 2.7 million Americans infected with a liver disease, known as hepatitis C. One of the most noticeable areas of divergence between alternative and conventional protocols is found in the treatment of such liver disorders. I will compare the treatments. You may be surprised to see the alternative approach, which is much more conservative, can be quite effective.

Conventional treatment of Hepatitis C

The available information supplied by the manufacturers of the conventional medications (alpha interferon family) presently used in the treatment of Hepatitis C states that the response rate was about 30 percent. At the same time, I noticed clinical trials listed on the sites indicated side effects of fatigue/asthenia occurred in 65 percent, and headache at 43 percent. In addition, other, much more serious adverse events occurred at lesser levels. The manufacturer's website listed about a 20 percent rate of psychiatric adverse events. In addition, the Rebetrol website disclosed severe psychiatric adverse events, depression, along with "suicidal behavior, (suicidal ideation, suicidal attempts and suicides) have occurred during combination Rebetol/Intron A (REBETRON) therapy and with Interferon Alpha monotherapy, both in patients with and without a previous psychiatric illness."

Alternative Treatment of Hepatitis C

Burt Berkson, M.D. Ph.D., recalls his first experience in treating advanced liver disease over 27 years ago. At that time, Berkson was an internist who was asked to make two patients comfortable as they were expected to die as a result of their advanced liver failure. Berkson treated the patients using intravenous alpha lipoic acid. Within two weeks the liver patients recovered and he states he was called on the carpet for having used the natural anti-oxidant. Medical experts referred to the incident as "spontaneous recovery," an unexplained case of total recovery. One week later Berkson again, treated two more patients in the last stages of liver failure with intravenous alpha lipoic acid. The two patients recovered. The story gets better.

In a 1999 Abstract published in PUBMED Berkson reports: "…The triple antioxidant combination of alpha-lipoic acid, silymarin and selenium was chosen for a conservative treatment of hepatitis C because these substances protect the liver from free radical damage, increase the levels of other fundamental antioxidants, and interfere with viral proliferation. The three patients presented in this paper followed the triple antioxidant program and recovered quickly and their laboratory values remarkably improved. Furthermore, liver transplantation was avoided and the patients are back at work, carrying out their normal activities, and feeling healthy. The author offers a more conservative approach to the treatment of hepatitis C that is far less expensive. One year of the triple antioxidant therapy described in his paper costs less than $2,000, as compared to more than $300,000 a year for liver transplant surgery. "It appears reasonable, that prior to liver transplant surgery evaluation, or during the transplant evaluation process, the conservative triple antioxidant treatment approach should be considered. If there is a significant betterment in the patient's condition, liver transplant surgery may be avoided." By the way, silymarin is also known as milk thistle, long known for its ability to promote liver health.

This almost sounds like an urban legend except that in looking for background on Berkson, I found that Berkson was a principal Food & Drug Administration (FDA) investigator in the use of intravenous alpha lipoic acid, consultant to the National Institutes of Health (NIH) as well as consultant for the Centers for Disease Control and Prevention (CDC).

Will his treatment work for all cases of Hepatitis C? Perhaps not, but remember chances of conventional therapy being effective run in the 30 percentile range, based on information supplied by manufacturers of alpha interferon products. Additionally, the side effects of the conventional "cures" are abundant. The more natural, conservative treatment is certainly worth looking into and anyone interested in Dr. Berkson's approach to treatment can contact him at the Center for Integrative Medicine, 741 N. Alameda Blvd. Las Cruces, New Mexico 88005. Phone: 505-524-3720. You may also learn more by purchasing Berkson's publication: The Alpha Lipoic Acid Breakthrough. The administration of Dr. Berkson's intravenous treatment must be performed by a health professional.

Immune system: Delta-Immune—Amazing immune support

The horrifying Chernobyl nuclear power plant disaster that claimed the lives of over 20,000 people created urgency for Russian research scientists. Out of the disaster came a discovery that has proven effective in protecting the immune system, according to Dr. Robert Jay Rowen's March 2005 newsletter, *Second Opinion*. Rowen discussed the Russian discovery and its growing use in the United States over the last five years.

The Russian government sought scientists who would work to find something that might help mitigate the radiation poisoning the Chernobyl victims suffered. Russian and Bulgarian microbiologists had already been working on protection against biological warfare agents so were somewhat prepared for working in the direction of a solution to radiation poisoning.

The finished product was similar to what we know as a probiotic (friendly bacteria in the intestines), however, the new product contained no live bacteria but rather supplied the intestinal walls with proteins that supported natural immune response. The discovery worked by creating an environment that promoted friendly intestinal bacterial growth. The product was called Delta-Immune or Russian Choice Immune.

Why should intestinal bacteria be viewed with such importance?

Dr. Rowen explains in his newsletter that the majority of the body's immune cells are located in the intestinal tract. The Russian/Bulgarian product was made from a specific strain of lactobacillus rhamnosus. The scientists developed a process that penetrated or fractured the cell walls of the lactobacillus, creating potent cell wall fragments that turned out to be much stronger than acidophilus in creating an effective immune system. A strong immune system response is needed to fight off both infections and diseases.

Most of us are aware that the live bacteria in acidophilus is necessary for proper digestion and as an assistant to the immune system. The new product and its cell fragment function, however, were quite dissimilar from basic acidophilus. The new immune booster acted in a synergistic manner in promoting a healthy intestinal environment.

Dr. Rowen stated that the first tests on the product were conducted on mice that had been irradiated. By day seven, those mice treated with the Delta-Immune, possessed six times the antibody production as the control group mice. The substance was administered to victims of Chernobyl with positive results, according to Rowen.

The most interesting aspect of this product is that it is helpful for many disorders, including bronchitis, according to Rowen. That is frequently the case with nutrients. Most nutrients and natural foods that are good for one part of the system, also complement other parts of the system.

The product is sold under numerous names, Del-Immune, Delta Immune and Russian Choice Immune. It was first sold in the US by Nutricology and now is being sold by several companies under various names. To learn more about Delta-Immune you can call Nutricology at 800-545-9960 or Vital Nutrients at 877-747-9139. These are only a few of the companies that sell the product.

As always, speak with your own physician about this or any other complementary supplements you may be considering.

KIDNEY AND GALL STONES—RAIN FOREST WONDER CHANCA PIEDRA—

For those who suffer kidney stones, there may be hope in the form of an herb from the rain forests that has been shown to be effective in dissolving the painful culprits. The herb is known as chanca piedra—translated, "stone breaker" or "shatter stone." It may also be helpful in the treatment of gallstones. Detailed information on the herb is explained in a new book, *The Healing Power of Rainforest Herbs* by Leslie Taylor. The book explains the usage of over 70 botanicals grown in the rainforests that are used by indigenous peoples for healing. The chanca piedra plant comes from the Phyllanthus (niruri, amarus) genus of the herb family that contains 600 species. Not all of the species are effective in doing the job of breaking stones and unfortunately, the names are sometimes used interchangeably, which has created problems among researchers in identifying the correct species for use in clinical trials. The chanca piedra plant has a long history of use in the Amazon and other tropical regions where it is grown, as an herbal medicine. The book explains the analysis of the plant. It has been found to be rich in lignans, glycosides, flavonoids, phenylpropanoids, and ellagitannins. These may not mean much to the average person, but they are all beneficial to the system in one form or another.

The book reports on various studies of the herb. In 1990, the Paulista School of Medicine in San Paulo, Brazil conducted studies on humans, rats and mice. It was used in the form of a tea for up to three months and the results showed the herb dissolved stones. In one 1999 in vitro study, the herb inhibited the formation of calcium oxalate crystals that cause kidney stones. The 42-day study indicated that chanca piedra worked to inhibit the formation of stones among the control group with several of the animals passing the stones. It has also been used as an anti-spasmodic agent in cases of kidney stones. Because of this "relaxing" effect, it is not recommended for pregnant women. Another 2000 study documented that the product increased the life span of control group mice. According to the literature, it has a liver protective quality that may be the result of those strange named above properties.

While studies and application of the herb in other countries are showing great promise, it is not an herb one would take without the assistance of a health professional. It is strong. It would have to be to dissolve stones. It has been known to decrease blood pressure and is also used in the tropics to treat hypertension. However, that may pose a problem for people with existing low blood pressure or those on blood pressure medications because it potentiates (makes stronger) the effects of blood pressure medication. It is especially not recommended for those on drugs known as ACE inhibitors such as Altace. Additionally, it possesses a diuretic effect.

In reading the information available on chanca piedra, it is clear the rainforest herb contains many healthful substances and shows great promise for use in liver disorders as well as for kidney stones and kidney stone prevention along with possible use for gallstones. If something in the plant is patentable, it may well be used by pharmaceuticals in the treatment of stones and other disorders, however, should there be no patentable qualities, we will have to wait for more human research. The book is excellent but it is important to remember that any substance can have contraindications that one might not be aware of. It is important to notify your physician of any supplements or herbs you may be taking.

The book can be purchased at Amazon.com for $16.95 or at Barnes & Noble for $15.95.

The informative book reminds us that the rainforests are indeed, healing places that provide us with protection. This protection works both ways.

LITHIUM: A PROTECTION FOR THE BRAIN?

I truly believe that God has created a cure for every disease known to man. The problem is to find those cures and to learn to develop habits and lifestyles that will help us prevent the disease process itself. I subscribe to the top alternative newsletters in the country and abroad. Many times the research is years ahead of the curve and of an informative and simple nature, I enjoy passing the data along to readers—hopefully—to enable them to work with their own physicians to further research various newer and more natural methods that might be useful in assisting them in the treatment of various conditions.

The Tahoma Washington Clinic of Dr. Jonathan Wright is to alternative medicine what the "Mayo Clinics" is to conventional medicine. He recently wrote about the benefits of a little known but valuable mineral from the sodium and potassium family. The mineral is lithium. Dr. Wright points out that in the 1930's and 1940's, lithium was sold over the counter as a salt substitute until it was realized that too much lithium could be toxic.

Dr. Wright has noted that there are many uses for low-dose lithium for both brain protection, and to treat mental disorders as well-being helpful in treating other physical disorders. Some alternative physicians believe lithium has not been used more widely because it is a simple mineral and cannot be patented by any pharmaceuticals.

I clearly remember, in the early 1970's, a radio news report claiming an agency within the federal government had placed lithium into the El Paso, Texas water supply to test its efficacy against violent crimes and other violent behavior. Indeed, crime rates dropped, as did other violent behavior. I personally, was livid over the thought that the government could take such license without the permission of the citizens of that town. Throughout the years, we have learned that our government conducted such experiments, some brutal, which resulted in taxpayers being forced to pay punitive damages to unknowing victims of such experimentation. The study showed that lithium had a calming effect.

Dr. Wright also explained that in cases of lithium toxicity, patients were able to mitigate the damage by taking flaxseed oil and a vitamin E supplement. The essential fatty acids in these supplements appear to resolve the problem of toxicity, according to the doctor. He explained his Tahoma Clinic physicians were treating a bi-polar patient who was on high dose lithium. According to Wright, the lithium worked well, but the patient began to show symptoms of toxicity (hypertension, tremor, nausea and protein in the urine). It was discovered that when she was given vitamin E oil along with flaxseed oil, her symptoms of toxicity disappeared. He now recommends that any of his patients on high-dose lithium supplement with flaxseed oil and vitamin E. Other interesting observations by Dr. Wright were that a report in Lancet, a British medical publication, indicated that, "Wayne State University (Detroit) researchers found that lithium has the ability to both protect and renew brain cells. Eight of 10 individuals who took lithium showed an average 3 percent increase in brain grey matter in just four weeks. Lithium may help to generate entirely new cells too: Another group of researchers recently reported that lithium also enhances nerve cell DNA replication. DNA replication is a first step in the formation of a new cell of any type."

Wright further states, "The Wayne State study used high-dose lithium, but I'm certainly not using that amount myself, nor do I recommend it. Prescription quantities of lithium just aren't necessary for 'everyday' brain cell protection and re-growth. Studies done years ago have shown that very low amounts of lithium can also measurably influence brain function for the better."

Wright has explained that low-dose lithium has been shown to control gout and to help in relieving some rashes caused by seborrheic dermatitis. He believes that once the positive benefits of low-dose lithium for brain protection become more widely known within the conventional medical community, the mineral will perhaps have application in reducing the progression of degenerative diseases such as Alzheimer's dementia and Parkinson's.

Dr. Wright's newsletter, Nutrition & Healing, also allows subscribers to take advantage of past medical reports and research via his website at wrightnewsletter.com. You can visit his Tahoma Clinic website at www.tahoma-clinic.com.

You may want to request your physician research the latest findings on lithium. Always discuss taking any supplement with your physician.

LYME DISEASE—THE GREAT IMITATOR—IMITATES MS, ALS

A number of years ago, in a small rural region of Connecticut, there was a mysterious outbreak of juvenile rheumatoid arthritis. When clusters of patients with a particular disease appear in any specific region, the Centers for Disease Control and Prevention (CDC) attempts to check it out. Several years later, the cause of the disease was discovered. A type of corkscrew-shaped bacteria known as a spirochete was found to be the culprit. As organisms, spirochetes are treacherous. The community was near Lyme, Connecticut, and as you may have guessed, the disease became known as "Lyme disease." It was then discovered to have been associated with deer ticks and a wildlife environment. Today, several high-profile alternative physicians seem to be concerned about newer developments regarding Lyme disease.

Recently, Dr. Robert Jay Rowen wrote of his special interest in the case of 34-year-old, Tom Coffey, who was believed to have Parkinson's disease and was eventually diagnosed with ALS (Lou Gehrig's disease). The young man had lost his ability to swallow and was fed through a feeding tube. He was given a life expectancy of months and sent home from the hospital. The young man, not willing to give up, had nutritional support placed in his feeding tube. The added supplements seemed to improve his health. This surprised his doctors, since that was not a typical response in cases of ALS.

Coffey then remembered in recent months, having had a bull's eye rash that subsequently resolved. He remembered reading that the bull's eye rash was a sign of the Lyme tick bite and saw a Lyme disease specialist who placed him on the antibiotic Rocephin. Amazingly, he recovered and his story appeared in "People Magazine."

Dr. Rowen believes that even more recent findings indicate there is a great chance that conventional medicine may be overlooking Lyme disease as a cause of many symptoms and diseases, not generally believed to be associated with Lyme. Lyme is difficult to detect and can mimic and cause many diseases, according to Rowen. He reports there are 300 conditions associated with this spirochete bacteria: Among the conditions are ALS, Parkinson's Disease, Alzheimer's disease, MS, fibromyalgia, muscle fatigue, rashes; coronary artery disease, Lupus, SIDS, and almost any inflammatory degenerative disease.

The spirochete from Lyme disease can corkscrew into muscle, tendons, ligaments and organs, according to Rowen. Infectious disease specialist, and victim of the disease, Joanne Whitaker, M.D. calls Lyme "the New Great Imitator" because of its insidious ability to cause symptoms of so many diseases.

Testing for Lyme disease is not that easy. Neither of the two available tests is deemed totally effective in diagnosing Lyme. The tests seek antibodies that may not always be present in the host's blood. The Lyme bug can hide so well, it may not show up on the tests. The CDC has set certain parameters to make a positive diagnosis; however, some patients are outside the parameters, yet have been found to have contracted Lyme disease. The CDC admits there is under-reporting of the disease. To add to the confusion, Dr. Rowen points to the case of a woman whose entire family showed up positive for Lyme disease, yet none of the family members had any association with a tick bite.

Rowen cites the findings of Wayne State University professor, Lida Mattman, PhD. Mattman states she found the presence of Lyme factor in hundreds of patients with any number of other diseases than Lyme disease. She also reports she found the Lyme spirochetes in mosquitoes and fleas as well as in human body fluids. Mattman's findings, according to Rowen, may well explain why entire families can become infected with this newly discovered disease—even in the absence of a tick bite. He believes Matman's profound discovery may be as great a revelation as the discovery that led to the identification of Lyme disease in the 1990's.

New Test—New Treatment

Now comes some good news. Dr. Joanne Whitaker, has developed a test that appears to actually detect the Lyme bug, not just the antibodies. Her test is known as Q-RIBb (quantitative rapid identification of Lyme disease, which scientifically carries the name Rb).

The news gets even better. It has been recently discovered that in those hard to treat cases, there is an herb that has been found effective against the Lyme disease spirochete. Because the herb works so well, it can create a reaction that quickly kills off the bug creating what is known as Herxheimer's (die off), which can cause reactions. Those who suspect their MS or other autoimmune disease may possibly be associated with Lyme, should contact a physician who is familiar with the new treatment and is willing to work with the patient to monitor the patient's progress. I will share more information on the disease, the herb and list some physicians who treat it. I will also give information on Dr. Whitaker's test and how readers can obtain more information on all of the above.

According to Dr. Robert Jay Rowen, "…this story will rock the very pillars of the medical establishment." Rowen is concerned that this insidious disease has a pervasive nature that allows it to "hide out" defying detection for as long as it wishes to wreak havoc on the immune system. Rowen believes that since Lyme disease is a relatively new medical discovery, the devastating nature of the disease has yet to be understood by the general medical community. He points to the discovery by researcher Lida Mattman, PhD., that the Lyme spirochete had been detected in mosquitoes, ticks, fleas and body fluids.

Dr. Rowen explains that the present parameters for diagnosing Lyme as well as the tests currently available are sorely lacking and may well fail to spot many additional cases of Lyme infection.

On the upside, Rowen points to the promising news that infectious disease specialist, Dr. Joanne Whitaker, has developed a newer test that actually detects the Lyme bug itself, rather than antibodies which may elude detection.

Dr. Whitaker's belief that Lyme is "The New Great Imitator" may explain how so many cases may be misdiagnosed. Dr. Rowen states: "there have been a number of patients who appear to be legitimately diagnosed with autoimmune diseases when in fact, they had Lyme disease." Many of those patients have either recovered or greatly improved when treated for Lyme disease.

In no way is this recent revelation, meant to suggest that every patient diagnosed with autoimmune diseases, actually has Lyme disease. In fact, Rowen clearly states that Lyme may merely be an opportunistic disease that attacks an already compromised immune system. The point the alternative physicians are making is that checking for Lyme with the newer test developed by Dr. Whitaker, may help eliminate the possibility of Lyme, being the underlying cause of some autoimmune diseases. He also believes that legitimate immune disorders may be exacerbated by the presence of the Lyme spirochete and, if detected with the new test, should be treated.

Rowen points to Tom Coffey, who was incorrectly diagnosed first with MS and then with Lou Gehrig's disease and sent home to die after his condition deteriorated. Coffey remembered a bull's-eye rash from a tick bite and sought a Lyme disease specialist. He totally recovered after being treated for Lyme disease.

In those cases where conventional protocol did not help patients with Lyme disease, an herb called "cat's claw" was effectively administered, according to Rowen. Please note the herb found in health food stores is not in the proper form. It must be purchased as TOA-free cat's claw.

Rowen further writes of the case of Larry Powers, a former Mr. America competition winner, who was diagnosed with Parkinson's disease and confined to a wheel chair. After hearing about the Lyme connection to Parkinson's, Powers obtained TOA-free cat's claw and after three weeks of cautious use, became ambulatory.

Important note about MS

Dr. Mattman's studies have also shown that L-form bacteria is present in inflamed tissue, a common finding among MS patients. She believes that while this particular bacterium is not associated with Lyme disease, it too can invade the central nervous system to cause chronic inflammation that may lie at the root of MS. Because L-form bacteria has no cell wall structure, it is able to evade detection. However, a conventional antibiotic, Minocycline, seems to work against the stealth bacteria. Dr. Robert Jay Rowen says it is used to treat MS relapse.

Conventional medicine is beginning to adopt the theory and treatment.

Dr. Rowen does not recommend any patient self-treat because of the rapid die-off of toxins. It is important to seek out a physician who will test and treat for Lyme and the possibility of L-form among MS patients.

A cardiologist, who treats difficult cases of Lyme with TOA-free cat's claw along with nutrition, is Dr. Lee Cowden of Fort Worth, Texas. He uses a strict nutritional protocol and closely monitors each of his patients.

If you feel you would like to further research this new development because you believe you may have contracted Lyme, ask your physician to contact Bowen Laboratories to obtain the new test. The new test cannot be administered without a physician's referral and all reports will be sent to your physician. If you do not have a physician who is interested, Bowen Labs maintains a database of referring physicians who will administer the test for you. The test may be obtained by calling 727-937-9077.

IBS—helped by TOA-free cat's claw

Dr. James Balch author of the newsletter *Prescriptions for Healthy Living,* writes in his March 2005 issue TOA-free cat's claw as being helpful in treating yet other more common intestinal disorder prevalent among Americans, Irritable Bowel Syndrome or IBS. He states it may also be useful for treating Crohn's disease and gastritis. Dr. Balch states some patients have recovered after years of suffering by using the particular form of samento that has been used to treat Lyme disease. He states that in Peru, cat's claw tea is said to have "unlimited curative properties."

Balch is unsure of exactly why the treatment is effective; however, he opines that it may be that IBS sufferers have a hidden infection. Samento has some powerful anti-infection properties. Samento contains quinovic acid glycosides which are natural quinolones, but much safer than antibiotics such as Cipro, according to Dr. Balch.

Drs. Balch and Rowen both warn that in order for cat's claw herb to be effective, it must be labeled TOA-free. It goes through a process that removes the TOA portion that inhibits the agents that kill bacteria. When TOA is removed, the other agents are strong and can work to fight bacteria. Both Balch and Rowen give sources for obtaining TOA-free cat's claw as Nutricology, Prima Una de Gata and Nutramedix. This is a very new find and your physician may not be aware of it. This does not mean that every case of MS or ALS is caused by the Lyme bug or can be treated with TOA-free cat's claw.

LUPUS—FISH OIL IS IMPORTANT

Once again, good news about improving the symptoms of a disease without drastic drugs comes very simple. The disease: Lupus. The answer: fish oil. Lupus, is an insidious disease in which the body's immune system attacks the body's own organs. It can result in swollen joints, fatigue, skin rashes and kidney or heart problems. Unfortunately, many times it begins to show up at the tender age of 30 and strikes mostly young women. The cause of Lupus is yet unknown. Lupus affects 40 to 50 people per 100,000.

While fish oil is not a cure, it has been shown in a study reported by the British Broadcasting Corporation, to be helpful in reducing the symptoms of Lupus by reducing inflammation naturally. It is believed the fatty acids found in the fish oil act as an anti-inflammatory agent.

The six-month study involved patients with active Lupus and the participants were given either fish oil three times per day, copper, or copper plus fish ol or a placebo. The copper was of no benefit, however, all of the patients taking fish oil had improvement in inflammation and fatigue, according to the report. The improvements ranged from mild to drastic. NOTE: I might also state here that those with immune diseases such as Lupus should never take the immune booster echinacea. Echinacea may easily exacerbate the condition making the wayward immune system stronger and more able to attack the body.

Presently, there are several drugs, including steroids that are used to treat Lupus. However, these are not without side effects, which can sometimes add to the discomfort of the condition itself. During the study, some of the participants took fish oil along with their steroids and according to the researchers, were able to reduce the amount of steroids they were taking.

Dr. Joseph Mercola often writes about the important benefits of fish oils especially for children. Both fish oil and cod liver oil contain essential fatty acids DHA and EPA). The types of fat in fish and cod liver oil is known as omega 3 and omega 6. Both are necessary components of health, however, the American diet contain an imbalance in the two and Mercola states we ingest too much omega 6. Dr. Mercola states, "The primary sources of omega-6 are corn, soy, canola, safflower and sunflower oil; these oils are overabundant in the typical diet, which explains our excess omega-6 levels. Avoid or limit these oils. Omega-3, meanwhile, is typically found in flaxseed oil, walnut oil, and fish."

He further points out, "By far, the best type of omega-3 fats are those found in that last category, fish. That's because the omega-3 in fish is high in two fatty acids crucial to human health, DHA and EPA. These two fatty acids are pivotal in preventing heart disease, cancer, and many other diseases. The human brain is also highly dependent on DHA—low DHA levels have been linked to depression, schizophrenia, memory loss, and a higher risk of developing Alzheimer's. Researchers are now also linking inadequate intake of these omega-3 fats in pregnant women to premature birth and low birth weight, and to hyperactivity in children."

Mercola also points out that a problem with fish is avoiding fish with high mercury content. This is difficult since our oceans, lakes and streams are so polluted and fish become victims of their environment. One brand of mercury-free fish oil and cod liver oil that he recommends is Carlson products and Living Fuel. He also recommends using caution in eating mercury-laden fish and suggests a company called Vital Choice to purchase mercury-free salmon.

Dr. Mercola recommends that because of the high Vitamin D content in cod liver oil, it be consumed in the winter months, while fish oil be taken in the summer months in order to avoid too much vitamin D.

MAMMOGRAM VS. THERMOGRAPHY

There is no doubt in my mind that the person(s) who invented the Mammogram have at least a distant relationship to the Marquis de Sade. I once had a mammogram. I once had a trash compactor. Same concept.

On the more serious side, there are questions being raised about the effectiveness of mammography as well as differences in the radiological interpretations. There are also questions about the effects of the radiation as well as possible effects of the mechanical pressure of the Mammogram releasing small, encapsulated cancers. There is debate on exactly what age group would be helped by Mammography and hopefully, the "experts" will be able to define the efficacy of Mammograms sooner than they were able to determine that hormone replacement therapy wasn't exactly a good idea.

I've been reading about another screening tool recommended by alternative physicians for detecting breast problems including infection and cancers. The system is known as thermography. The concept of thermography is that heat is generated from inflammation within the breast when the cancer or infectious process is taking place. Thermography is so heat-sensitive that it picks up any inflammation process much earlier than other screening tools. There is no radiation exposure involved in thermography. It detects the growth of new blood vessels that are formed by tumors. Thermography can detect even the smallest of changes in breast temperature. Alternative physicians feel this is beneficial in that specific dietary intervention can be implemented to help strengthen the body's immune response.

I was so interested in thermography that I decided to learn more about the system by contacting several physicians who use thermography as a screening tool. Thermography was approved by the Federal Drug Administration (FDA) for use in screening for breast cancer, vascular disease of the lower extremity (deep vein thrombosis), extra cranial blood vessel disease and neuro-musculoskeletal problems. The problem appears to be that there are only a few hundred physicians around the country who are trained to use the rather inexpensive screening tool. The actual process was developed in 1957 and has become more perfected as technology advances. The numbers of physicians trained to use the equipment are growing, however, in my search for thermographic centers in Illinois there were only a few and none were in the Chicago area.

California chiropractor, William Cockburn, has studied thermography for many years and is presently training physicians throughout the U.S. in use of the non-invasive screening procedure.

One of Cockburn's major concerns is that there is no uniformity demanded in specifications for thermographic equipment. Patients presently must do their own research to see if the equipment used, is supported by the latest technology. "Some equipment out there is way behind the times and is being sold as the latest technology." Thermography is so new that guidelines are rather scant and Cockburn states that because there are so few experts on thermography, even physicians can be sold a bill of goods by a fast-talking salesman. Cockburn would like to see regulation and uniformity and has been part of a group lobbying for the establishment of specifications in thermography equipment. A good thermographic unit sells for about $50,000, which makes it even more appealing and cost-effective. The system has exciting medical possibilities and is being investigated as a screening tool for prostate cancer screening as well.

In all of my own research on various diseases, the common thread appears to be the inflammation process. Thermography has great potential in detecting the inflammation process; I can't help but believe it will be recognized soon as a tremendous screening tool in the future to detect even more disorders.

It's an exciting, non-invasive, method that applies no mechanical pressure to the breast. It's a newer approach that those who use it believe can detect the very earliest signs of changes in breast tissue. It's suggested that patients obtain a baseline thermography and then have one each year thereafter to compare changes.

I had the opportunity to interview Dr. William Hobbins a delightful Madison, Wisconsin thoracic surgeon who has used thermography as a screening tool since the early 1970's. I might add, that after speaking with this gifted sage, I came away with a far greater understanding of the fundamentals of both health and logic.

Dr. Hobbins states, "Thermography will become the new paradigm in breast screening." The confident 80-year young, physician went on to explain the protocol he has found most effective for treating early breast cancer formation. He noted that breast cancer begins about eight years prior to a physician or patient being able to palpate a dime-sized lump. He posits that in the early stages as breast cancer begins to form, a process known as angiogenesis takes place. Angiogenesis is the formation of new blood vessels around a tumor. The blood vessels form to help feed the tumor, enabling it to grow. This process then creates a "fever" in the breast, according to Hobbins. "Thermography is sensitive enough to pick up this "fever" long before Mammography will pick up a lump," explained Hobbins. Once he discovers the formation of these new blood vessels he then prescribes anti-angiogenesis agents to stop any further formation of blood vessels. He states that the early-stage tumor is starved to death because no "food" in the form of blood, can supply the tumor. He also says that earlier detection may result, at the most, in lumpectomies, not mastectomies and toxic chemotherapy. At times he uses other tools such as ultrasound and MRI in addition to thermography; however, I am focusing on his basic concept of thermography.

Hobbins is also unique in that, he provides his patients with a most informative health newsletter listing the latest in health news. Hobbins says there are problems with present methods of detecting and treating breast cancer. He sees Mammography as an inadequate screening tool. "Women of various ages have different types of breast tissue," says Hobbins. He goes so far as to say, "It is a crime for women under 50 to be subjected to Mammograms." He is surely not alone. In 1974, Professor Malcolm C. Pike at the University of Southern California School of Medicine advised the National Cancer Institute that specialists had concluded, "giving a women under age 50 a mammogram on a routine basis is close to unethical." In fact, this advice had been heeded until the 1980's.

Dr. Hobbins explained that mammography is only 41 percent sensitive in women under age 50, while ultrasound is 68 percent sensitive. There are also concerns about radiation when Mammograms are given on a yearly basis.

Sherrill Sellman, author of the book "*Hormone Heresy: What Women Must Know About Their Hormones*" quotes Samuel Epstein, M.D., Professor of Occupational and Environmental Medicine at the University of Illinois School of Public Health. Epstein notes, "There is clear evidence that the breast, particularly in premenopausal women, is highly sensitive to radiation, with estimates of increased risk of up to one percent for every RAD (radiation absorbed dose) unit of x-ray exposure. Even for low dosage exposure of two RADs or less, this exposure can add up quickly for women having an annual mammography."

Sellman also quotes another expert, Dr. Charles B. Simone, a former clinical associate in immunology and pharmacology at the National Cancer Institutes., "Mammograms increase the risk for developing breast cancer and raise the risk of spreading or metastasizing an existing growth," says the doctor. Sellman says, "Safer and even more effective diagnostic techniques like infrared thermography, has been vigorously attacked by the Breast Cancer Awareness organizations."

It's up to us to seek out the best care available and from what I've read, thermography is a start. Unfortunately, medicine can be very political, so those seeking thermography may find resistance from their physicians.

NOTE: Additionally, a study reported in the Journal of the National Cancer Institutes (January 2005) explains that a malfunction in the manner in which the body processes vitamin A may lead to cells becoming cancerous. Cell differentiation is the key, according to the article. Cell differentiation is what occurs when vitamin A is used by the breast as needed. When a malfunction in the ability of the body to express this differentiation occurs, the cells may become cancerous.

MARGARINE: VS. BUTTER: WE'VE BEEN MISLED

Anyone on the Internet knows about the "urban legends" that sail through the ether faster than a speeding bullet. I'm still getting forwarded emails urging me to send "get well" cards to 7 year old Craig Shergold—who happens to be about 35 years old by now.

There are all types of false medical alerts that circulate as well. I mostly delete the stuff until I received a forwarded email about margarine and its dangers. That one interested me because I knew most of the content of the email was accurate. I even checked out snopes.com and Lo! They give it credibility.

Years ago, the conventional medical community adopted a theory that margarine was more healthy than butter because it contained fewer grams of fat. Turns out it was a mistake. Margarines and many other foods that use a process known as "hydrogenation" are not healthy. The conventional community operated on the belief that margarine had fewer saturated fats (5 grams compared to butter's 8 grams) even though both had the same number of calories. However, it has what are known as "trans fats" or "trans fatty acids." These fats are exceptionally dangerous and the conventional medical community has only recently come around to understand the dangers of hydrogenation and trans fats.

I first read of the suspected problems with margarine in my son's copy of *Science Digest* in the early 1980's. The "Digest" wrote of the suspected dangers of hydrogenation. The hydrogenation process is what makes liquid oils into hard fats by changing a few molecules.

The article explained there was a question of whether the body could handle the hydrogenation process. Because the molecules were double-bonded, there was some concern that these fats would not leave the system and may actually accumulate. Medical science is beginning to understand the serious problem with hydrogenation. Hydrogenation is what makes your margarine spread, it makes the texture smooth. Hydrogenation stops foods from separating. Peanut butter is a prime example. In health food stores, the oil sits on top of the peanut butter and must be mixed as it is used. This is actually far healthier according to alternative physicians.

Butter, while it contains fat is actually healthier than margarine. Alternative physicians also suggest that if we must use butter, we must use it sparingly. They suggest we never use margarines.

We seem to operate in a world of confusion about types of fats. First the conventional medical community chased down saturated fats. That was one of the reasons they adopted the theory that margarine was better than butter. They never sought the whole picture.

The butter versus margarine issue is a prime example of how the medical community can go so wrong. For years doctors have been telling patients to replace butter with margarine. I did it only when I was baking cookies or cakes. Since cookies and cakes are no good for anyone, I figured the margarine I baked with wouldn't make a difference.

Another example of wrong-headed thinking was in the case of sounding the alarm on eggs. Eggs have lutein that you need for your vision. Eggs have fats but they also contain natural lecithin to counter the fats. The lecithin is most helpful when the eggs are soft boiled. Frying anything is unhealthy, including eggs.

One of the first to sound the alarm on hydrogenation was researcher Mary Enig. She fought the medical community head-on as she watched the American Heart Association overtake the American Medical Association (AMA) in demanding a new health policy be adopted that excluded butter and replaced it with margarine. The AMA was hesitant to adopt the policy many years ago but eventually fell into line adopting the medical mistake, according to Enig. Dr. Enig explains that trans fatty acids pose a danger to the heart and the entire immune system.

Enig says, "Basically, trans fatty acids cause alterations to numerous physiological functions of biological membranes that are known to be critical for cell homeostasis, e.g., appropriate membrane transport and membrane fluidity, and these fatty acid isomers produce alterations in adipose cell size, cell number, lipid class and fatty acid composition." You may not understand what she is saying, but basically she is elaborating on what *Science Digest* wrote of so many years ago. These phony fats are dangerous and according to Enig, actually interfere with the body's normal protective processes.

In alternative medicine a simple rule of thumb is that if it's natural it's most likely to be healthier. Butter is natural. Does it contain fats? Yes, it does. Is it a healthy food? Not necessarily because of the fats, but it's healthier than any margarines that are hydrogenated or partially hydrogenated.

MASTIC GUM: ANTIBACTERIAL FOR TEETH AND STOMACH

When I hear the word "mastic" it elicits visions of glue and sticky adhesive used in applying floor tiles, so when I heard of a "mastic" gum, it sounded quite unappealing. Masticha or Mastic, botanical, pistachia schinus-lentiscus is a resin derived from an evergreen bush in Greece. By its name one can see it is related to the pistachio tree family. It is grown on the Island of Chios.

It has been used for thousands of years as help for both stomach disorders and gingival protection in the Mediterranean region, Arabic countries and Western Europe, especially France. It's interesting that attempts have been made to grow it in other regions of the world with very little success. It would seem the Greeks have a natural patent on the substance.

It is always heartening to know that most natural healing substances are useful in promoting overall good health. For that reason, it isn't surprising to learn that a substance that supports gingival health can also be of assistance in treating digestive conditions such as ulcers.

There is growing evidence that reflux can be helped by chewing any sugar free gum (no aspartame) after meals. (The sugar free gum suggested was sweetened with Xylitol). Mastic gum provides additional benefits as a result of its anti-bacterial properties. In a Japanese study the group using mastic gum reduced gingival inflammation by 50 percent over the placebo group. Mastic has been proven to have an effect on a number of bacterium. That may explain why it has been so effective in treating bad breath. It is also interesting to learn that most of the research and written information on Masticha or Mastic, appears in foreign publications, especially in Europe where use of mastic is rapidly growing. There are very few American journals that have even referred to the resin. Considering all of the reading of research I do on a daily basis, I was surprised I hadn't heard of mastic until alternative physician Richard Becker, D.O. mentioned it on his television program. Also mentioned was Leo Galland, M.D., of New York. Both physicians speak of the use of mastic gum in the treatment of ulcers.

One particular type of bacteria associated with stomach ulcers is Helicobacter Pylori (H-pylori). Mastic has been found to kill at least seven forms of H-pylori bacteria along with a number of other bacterium that may account for its efficacy in treating ulcer conditions and other digestive discomforts. This very quality shows great promise in the treatment of ulcers, considering that much of the antibiotic therapy we presently use can prove futile due to the problem of bacteria becoming resistant to various antibiotic therapies. That is one of the problems we face today with the constant dispensing of antibiotics for every little cough and cold. Germs are smart and learn to mutate and become resistant to antibiotics. Mastic is unique in that it is not considered an antibiotic yet has proven to kill a great number of pathogens and has antioxidant properties because of its phenolic acid content. Another benefit of mastic was that it was shown in other studies to inhibit the growth of e-coli and staph as well as salmonella as well as some forms of fungus.

Leo Galland M.D., a physician who treats many patients with chronic gastric disorders in his New York practice, states he has effectively treated patients with intestinal permeability, ulcers, and dyspepsia through the use of mastic. In his own clinical trials, Dr. Galland used mastic in 500 mg. to one gram in capsule form twice a day for two weeks. He states after two weeks the H-pylori was eliminated in 80 percent of his patients, while 90 percent experienced symptomatic relief. Mastic is available in both gum and capsule form.

Both Dr. Becker and Dr. Galland believe mastic possesses stomach lining protective features while eliminating the H-pylori bacteria. The gum can be purchased as Emla MASTICgum at Life Enhancement at 1-800-543-3873. The capsules can be purchased at FUBAO Health by calling—1-866-883-8221, Herbal Nutrition at 1-888-294-6365 or online at iherb.com.

Chances are that your physician and dentist have never heard of mastic gum. It's a new one for me. It may be a good idea to ask your physician or other health care professional to research it for you.

MIGRAINE HEADACHES: A FEW VIEWS ON CAUSES AND TREATMENT

Part I of this chapter give a little background and poses the views of numerous alternative/conventional health professionals. **Part II** of this chapter contains the latest update that incorporates some of the measures from part one and adds additional findings and conclusions that resulted in a 100 percent cure rate of all subjects in the study.

Migraine headaches can be a most debilitating and crippling disorder. Migraines can bring even the strongest of men and women to tears; although migraines appear to occur more frequently among women. Some migraines are so severe; they can create double-vision, fainting and trips to the emergency room. There are numerous theories as to the cause of migraine headaches.

According to Schaumburg physician, Dr. Joseph Mercola, migraine headaches can be caused by sensitivities to various foods, such as wheat, dairy and especially sugars. He suggests that artificial sweeteners and even chemicals in foods can trigger migraine headaches. It is becoming apparent that stress may be a factor in the development or exacerbation of many existing diseases, including migraines.

An article appearing in *Life Extension Magazine* (February 2004) explains some of the latest research on migraines. The article, written by Romy Fox points to research that indicates the very conditions that deplete the body's magnesium stores, such as alcohol, stress and pregnancy may trigger migraine headaches. The article explains that, "Up to half of the people who suffer migraines are deficient in the free and active form of magnesium known as serum ionized magnesium. If free magnesium levels fall too low, the vessels supplying the blood to the head may 'clamp down' inappropriately, hindering blood flow in the head and triggering a migraine." He references the studies conducted by neurologist, Alexander Mauskop, a leading authority on migraines and author of *"What Your Doctor*

May Not Tell You About Migraines." In one Mauskop study, patients in the throes of migraine headaches who also showed low levels of free magnesium were given intravenous injections of magnesium, which halted their headaches—sometimes within 15 minutes.

Fox reports that Mauskop's study found that the lower the free magnesium among the migraine sufferers, the more quickly relief was felt, and the more long-lasting relief was realized after the magnesium injections. Even without injections, Dr. Mauskop felt that magnesium supplements would be helpful. The doctor's study explained that minor deficiencies in magnesium are widespread and that 15 to 20 percent of Americans "suffer from chronic magnesium deficiency." He recommends between 300 to 400 mg. of magnesium on a daily basis for those suffering migraine headaches.

Another possible help in the fight against the destructive headaches is riboflavin (vitamin B2) combined with magnesium. Riboflavin aids in the manufacture of red blood cells and assists in the creation of energy from carbohydrates, proteins and fats. Riboflavin (400 mg) alone yielded impressive results, but it took several months to prove effective. Additional studies have shown magnesium, riboflavin and the herbs feverfew and butterbur showed potential in relieving the painful condition.

The Fox article in *Life Extension* relates that in the 17th century, a British herbalist declared feverfew to be useful for "all pains in the head." Fox states both Britain and Canada have approved feverfew for use on migraine headaches. Studies are continuing to be conducted on the herbs as well as other supplements such as glucosamine, melatonin and Coenzyme Q10, all of which seem to show early signs of effectiveness in treating migraines. If medications don't seem to work, or you would rather try to obtain information on both conventional and natural treatment for migraines, you may be interested in the book by Dr. Mauskop "What Your Doctor May Not Tell You About Migraines."

Part II—Migraine update

A more recent study concluded in May of 2004, appears to offer a major breakthrough in treatment of migraine headaches. The conclusion of the six-month study has resulted in an astonishing success rate of 100 percent among the 21 women and two men in the study. That's truly phenomenal. Even more phenomenal is that the treatment within the study group also totally resolved every case of fibromyalgia, insomnia, depression and fatigue among the test group. That is just another benefit of treating causes rather than symptoms.

The newer research article authored by Dr. Sergey A. Dzugan, was written in the September 2004 issue of *Life Extension Magazine*. The study began at the North Central Mississippi Regional Cancer Center in Greenwood Mississippi, and was concluded at the Life Extension Foundation.

The latest hypothesis about migraine is that it is not one disorder but "…a specific consequence of the imbalance between neurohormonal and metabolic integrity." In other words, it is a "collection of disorders," which when addressed with the modalities used by the authors of the study, resulted in total relief for each of the participating migraine sufferers.

The new study uses many of the old findings and combines treatments to address each of the components. The successful multi-modality used by the researchers involved a four-part treatment. The first component was in creating a hormonorestorative therapy using bio-identical hormones that included a combination of oral pregnenolone, DHEA, triestrogen, progesterone and testosterone gels. The second part of the treatment involved correcting the imbalance between the sympathetic and parasympathetic nervous systems by balancing the ratio of calcium to magnesium. The third part of the treatment involved "resetting" of the pineal gland through melatonin supplementation. The fourth and seemingly unrelated, but necessary component was found in restoring the friendly intestinal flora with the use of quality probiotics.

The article explains, "Patients received treatment with oral pregnenolone, DHEA and dermal application of triestrogen (estriol 90%, estradiol 7%, estrone 3%, progesterone, and testosterone gels." This does not mean every patient should receive the same dosage. The treatment requires that first, specific serum hormone levels be obtained through a special type of test. As you can see, some parts of the hormonorestorative treatment were individualized and not administered on a one-size-fits-all scale; however, the melatonin was given in 3-6 mg. dosages while the magnesium was given in dosages of 420 mg. in the form of magnesium citrate.

The article points out that the study also included L-theanine or Kava root in the evening. Both are anti-anxiety agents. Kava is an herb and L-theanine is an amino acid derived from green tea. There is presently a debate about kava and its action on the liver, so the study allowed patients who were concerned about kava, to substitute with l-theanine.

The article becomes very technical and there are other variables involved which means that for those interested in this new treatment, a copy of the article should be obtained and given to your physician.

You can contact Life Extension at www. LEF.org.

NATTOKINASE—WONDER
ENZYME—PREVENTION OF BLOOD CLOTS?

There were glowing T.V. news reports about a new blood thinner that will be easier to use and has fewer side-effects than the old stand-by, Coumadin (warfarin). The report also commented that Coumadin was initially developed as a rat poison. The components in Coumadin caused rats to bleed to death. Medical researchers observed the anti-clotting properties and it was tweaked a bit and began its use as a blood thinner in humans in the 1950's. The new product, Exanta, may well be better than Coumadin. The AP report stated that Exanta (ximelagatran) "works by targeting one coagulation factor; warfarin affects many." This in itself is good news, but as the researchers from Public Citizen always warn us, we should be a bit more reluctant to try new medications until they have been on the market for a few years.

The AP article also related that the makers of the new medication sponsored the studies. Most times problems with newer medications aren't discovered until after those medications are broadly prescribed to patients. Baycol and Rezulin were but a few of the examples where laboratory testing found no problems, however, they proved fatal to some patients. Both products were approved by the Food and Drug Administration (FDA)—but managed to destroy a few livers and were hastily removed from the market only months after being heralded as life-saving, wonder drugs. Exanta may prove useful and effective against blood clotting in humans, but the medical community is ignoring natural products that can also safely prevent blood clots.

One such product is known as nattokinase (natto), which was first discovered by Japanese physician, Hiroyuki Sumi in 1980. Natto is a cheese-like food initially derived from soybeans, however, it is fermented and additional healthy bacteria are added to the product. Health-conscious Japanese citizens now consume it as part of their daily diet. (From what I've read, one must develop a taste for natto). In a 1986 study, Dr. Sumi reported that natto had the highest fibrin dissolving activity among 200 foods throughout the world. The properties of natto resemble plasmin. Plasmin dissolves the dangerous fibrin that causes blood clots. Fibrin can form protein strands that block blood vessels leading to heart attack and stroke. Physicians generally place patients who have experienced stroke or heart attack on fibrin dissolving drugs such as Coumadin (warfarin) or the newer drug, Plavix, which helps keep platelets from sticking together. Some doctors recommend an aspirin a day for everyone.

Fibrin is not all bad. Fibrin is also what helps our bodies to heal when we are cut or wounded. Fibrin plugs are created by our bodies to stop us from bleeding to death and their formation along wounds help start the healing process. Without any fibrin, we will have excessive bleeding.

I recently heard of research on natto by Portland Oregon physician, Martin Milner, from the Center for Natural Medicine. Dr. Milner conducted his research in conjunction with Dr. Kouhei Makise of the Imadeqawa Makise Clinica in Kyoto, Japan. After completion of their research project, Dr. Milner wrote "In all my years of research as a professor of cardiovascular and pulmonary medicine, natto and nattokinase represent the most exciting new development in the prevention and treatment of cardiovascular related diseases," He also stated, "We have finally found a potent natural agent that can thin and dissolve clots effectively, with relative safety and without side effects."

Dr. Milner also believes that natto can be taken safely on a daily basis to prevent hardening of the arteries. "In some ways, Milner says, nattokinase is actually superior to conventional clot-dissolving drugs. T-PAs (tissue plasminogen activators) like urokinase (the drug), are only effective when taken intravenously and often fail simply because a stroke or heart attack victim's arteries have hardened beyond the point where they can be treated by any other clot-dissolving agent. Nattokinase, however, can help prevent that hardening with an oral dose of as little as 100 mg a day."

Studies have shown that natto works faster than some of the present clot busters, and maintains its activity from 4 to 12 hours as opposed to urokinase (the drug), which activates for only 4 to 20 minutes. Natto is being seen as useful for both reducing blood pressure as well as preventing osteoporosis because it also contains vitamin K2. Vitamin K2 depletion is seen as one cause of osteoporosis. Alternative physicians believe, natto holds promise for many disorders and even some types of infection because of a component in it, known as di-picolinic acid, which has antibacterial effects. Many alternative physicians openly state they wouldn't consider allowing patients to have surgery without taking natto.

It is important to remember that if you are presently taking blood thinners, you must not take natto. You should talk it over with your doctor and see if he/she would like to research natto and perhaps think about having you try it.

Natto costs about $40.00 to $50.00 per month, while most pharmaceutical blood thinners are priced at over $120.00 per month. Sales of natto will not bring any company wealth because it can't be patented.

Natto can be found in some Asian communities as a cheese-like product which is even less expensive. It can be purchased in capsule form at the Tahoma Clinic 1-888-893-6878, or at NEEDS—1-800-634-1380; Pure—1800-860-

9583 or Supplemart as "Naticore" at 1-877-255-8482 or go to the web site: iherbs.com. NOTE: If you are on blood thinners, do not take natto.

OLIVE OIL: BETTER THAN BUTTER AND MARGARINE

It's truly a health windfall when we can receive mega-benefits from convenient foodstuffs, generally on hand in the kitchen, or easily accessible at the local grocery store. One of those foodstuffs is good old fashioned extra virgin olive oil. Just as in the case of the delicious raw pineapple, extra virgin olive oil has many therapeutic functions. Olive oil is most largely used in the Mediterranean region. Numerous studies have pointed to the use of olive oil as part of the reason heart disease is much more rare among those who maintain a Mediterranean diet. Olive oil almost exclusively replaces margarine and butter in the region. In all fairness, however, olive oil is not the only factor that makes the Mediterranean diet so superior. The Mediterranean diet does not include as much meat as Americans consume and is higher in vegetable consumption as well as far less sugar consumption than that consumed in the United States.

New England cardiologist, Stephen Sinatra, often refers to recent research from the University of Barcelona that appeared in the *European Journal of Clinical Nutrition*. The research found that daily ingestion of extra virgin olive oil increased blood levels of oleic acid, vitamin E, and phenolic compounds.

Olive oil blocks bad cholesterol

Dr. Sinatra says monounsaturated fatty acids and phenolic compounds assist in blocking the oxidation of low-density lipoproteins (LDL), which is our bad cholesterol. Extra virgin olive oil has some of the healthiest components and anti-aging as well as anti-cancer properties.

The doctor points to extra virgin olive oil as not only being good for the heart but as providing even additional support for the immune system because "As an immuno-modulating agent; olive oil can reduce inflammation. It does this by modifying the production of inflammatory cytokines (proteins produced primarily by white blood cells) and tissue necrosis factors which when left unchecked can damage your eyes, brain, heart and skin. Interrupting these two steps in the inflammation cycle may be why olive oil is so beneficial in terms of skin protection."

Olive oil is helpful both internally and externally in protecting the skin's integrity and structure by helping the skin to maintain moisture. It's all but impossible to pronounce all of the wonderful healing properties of olive oil, and I'm thankful I can merely spell them out. Oleuropein and hydroxytyrosol, are two of the beneficial and potent scavengers of damaging free radicals, in olive oil, according to Sinatra. They account for a great deal of its healing properties. When the doctor tells us our LDL is high, he/she might tell us that we should use extra virgin olive oil instead of those other spreads, to help block the oxidation that creates the inflammation. In August I wrote of the latest studies, indicating inflammation is believed to be what leads to coronary heart disease. It appears extra virgin olive oil helps stop that inflammation process. If one were to protect one's heart from oxidation of LDL, it would be a major step in preventing hardening of the arteries or atherosclerosis, according to Dr. Sinatra.

Blood pressure reduction with extra virgin olive oil

A Spanish study has also shown that blood pressure can be reduced when olive oil is used to replace margarine, which contains hydrogenated fats. In both humans and animals (rats), olive oil was found to have relaxed the aorta and helped to reduce blood pressure. (So, who cares if rats have high blood pressure?)

Colon help with olive oil?

According to Dr. Sinatra, even more recent studies from 28 countries and four continents have demonstrated regular use of extra virgin olive oil was associated with reductions in colo-rectal cancers.

Of course, you really don't want to smother anything in olive oil, specifically because it is high in calories. While the fat in olive oil is good fat, even 14 grams of good fat per tablespoon, will plump you up like a balloon, so he recommends small daily doses of no more than 2 tablespoons at any one time.

Dr. Sinatra claims extra virgin olive oil is also helpful to the pancreas in that it doesn't cause the body to produce insulin as carbohydrates do.

By the way, in case you were curious about the name Sinatra; he says, indeed, he is a distant relative of the late famous crooner with the same name.

PLAVIX: *WORST PILLS/BEST PILLS* AUTHORS CITE NEW STUDY OF ITS DANGERS

This one really hit home. I collapsed onto the sofa, exhausted, apprehensive and in a daze. I had just returned home after visiting my husband at the hospital. I was wracking my brain trying to figure out what could have caused the excessive bleeding that landed him in the emergency room. He had no pain. No symptoms, just lots of lower intestinal blood loss. Before his stay was over, he required two units of blood to bring his dwindling blood count up from 8.5.

It bothered me because he had no signs or symptoms other than bleeding. He is among a group of patients who had been placed on Plavix long-term rather than the initial 30 to 60 days most physicians once prescribed.

In 2002, my 61-year old husband suffered what doctors described as a mild stroke. The extremely aggressive treatment and subsequent "piling on" of drugs and blood thinners, culminated into a nightmare resulting in a serious GI bleed that sent him slipping into shock and kidney failure. The trauma to his system exacerbated the symptoms of his stroke. Thankfully, he was stabilized and his kidney function returned.

As an avid reader *of Worst Pills/Best Pills*, I knew that many of the drugs he was prescribed while hospitalized in 2002 were not recommended by the authors of the publication—and were in fact, deemed dangerous. Have you ever attempted to question such protocols? Good luck. I did all I could humanly do including begging them to stop the parade of drugs, especially the blood thinners. In 2002, he had to be rushed in for endoscopic surgery to repair a gastrointestinal bleed. They then placed him on Plavix, ostensibly, to avoid another GI bleed.

So you can see, this new bleeding situation in March of 2005 had me worried. This time the bleed was not from the upper GI area but from the lower GI tract. I questioned whether the Plavix could have contributed to the bleed. It's a fairly new drug and there is not much data out there on its long-term use. He's been on it for three years.

My question was about to be answered, at least in part. As I perused the pile of mail I had avoided for several days, I opened my March issue of *Worst Pills/Best Pills* and on page 19, there was part of the answer in glaring headlines: **"Serious GI Toxicity With the Heart Drug Clopidogrel (PLAVIX)"** The issue related research that had been published in *the New England Journal of Medicine*, January 2005 issue. The research indicated Plavix was not safer, but rather, had a higher incidence of bleeding than aspirin. How timely. The *Worst Pills/Best Pills* articles explained: "The study was conducted to answer the question as to whether clopidogrel is a proper alternative to aspirin plus an antiulcer/heartburn drug, in this case esomeprazole for patients at high risk of developing an ulcer." Clopidogrel is Plavix. Esomeprazole is Nexium.

The study referenced by the authors of WP/BP indicated an "astonishingly high rate" of bleeding ulcers among patients taking clopidogrel (PLAVIX) as opposed to those taking aspirin along with esomeprazole (NEXIUM), an anti-ulcer drug.

The very situation the medication had promised to prevent was occurring in front of our eyes. The article related a change in stance by the authors of *Worst Pills/Best Pills*. They originally recommended clopidogrel be used only in patients who could not tolerate aspirin because of ulcers caused by aspirin or in cases of severe allergies to aspirin. The authors now state, "The only role that appears to be left for clopidogrel is in patients who have a severe allergy to aspirin."

In essence, the formerly accepted theory that clopidogrel is better for preventing bleeds is quite flawed, and the use of clopidogrel is not recommended by the authors except in cases of those who are allergic to aspirin.

The new study suggests that aspirin along with a drug from the proton pump inhibitor family (Prilosec, Nexium, Protonix, Aciphex, Nexium and their generic forms,) appear to be more effective than Plavix in preventing gastrointestinal bleeds.

If the results of this randomized controlled trial are to be accepted, it means many of us will save money. The authors recommend you speak to your doctor about switching back to low dose aspirin if you have no aspirin allergies. We pay $160.00 for a one-month supply of Plavix as opposed to about $1.50 for low-dose aspirin. We intend to bring the latest study to our physician. I believe Worst Pills/Best Pills is the first line of self-defense in protecting individuals from over-dosing with dangerous drugs. For those who do not have open-minded physicians, you may purchase Worst Pills/Best Pills newsletter by sending a check for $20.00 for one year or $36.00 for a two-year subscription to: Public Citizen, 1600 20th Street, NW; Washington, DC 20009. Make your check out to "Pill News" so they will know it's for the subscription. It's a worthy investment.

Power wash your arteries with Pomegranate Juice

One of my parent's favorite vocalists was a woman by the name of Rosemary Clooney. One of Clooney's songs was written by David Seville of Chipmunk fame. It was called "Come on-A My House." In one verse Clooney sang, "Come

on-a my house, I'm going to give you a marriage ring and a pomegranate too."
Can you believe that?

It seems Clooney was onto something with that pomegranate.

The pomegranate is coming of age lately. The red juice is chock full of phenolic acid, polyphenols and flavonoids. The juice also contains a rare fatty acid, punicic acid that is similar to conjugated linolenic acid (CLA). But there's much more to this delicious natural antioxidant drink. In fact, the antioxidant power of pomegranate juice is even superior to the antioxidant power of green tea.

The most recent scientific study available, while small, has confirmed previous study findings that showed pomegranate juice is effective in reversing arterial blockages by 30 percent. The Israeli study was conducted over a three-year period in which patients consumed the drink for three consecutive years. Measurements were taken at three-month intervals. The positive effects began showing up almost immediately. Other studies have shown pomegranate juice to reduce blood pressure slightly. Similar studies to that of the three-year study when conducted in mice have shown a 44% reduction in arterial plaque.

Dr. David Williams writes of the pomegranate in his May 2005 newsletter where he discusses research conducted at Rambam Medical Center in Haifa, Israel. The three-year study resulted in pomegranate juice showing a remarkable ability to affect and reverse artery blockage.

Williams quotes Dr. Michael Aviram of the Lipid Research Laboratory at Rambam, in Haifa, as stating that many high-risk heart patients may be spared bypass surgery merely by consuming pomegranate juice on a daily basis. The study involved 19 patients, 5 women and 14 men. Ten received about 8 ounces of 100 percent pomegranate juice daily, 9 of the patients were given a placebo. The primary test used to measure changes in the thickness of the carotid arteries was an ultrasound. After one year the non-pomegranate use group had an increase of 9 percent in thickness of the carotid, while those in the pomegranate group showed a decrease in thickness of 35 percent. The first three months of the study showed the pomegranate users with a 13 percent reduction in carotid wall thickness.

Williams points out that the pomegrante juice drinkers "had lower blood levels of oxidized cholesterol and more antioxidants. (*Clin Nutr 04;23:423-433*)."

Of course, there is always the problem of sugar in just about any juices we consume and this would have an impact on diabetics. Additionally, it is important to obtain pure pomegranate juice, not sweetened. I purchase it at local health food stores. It is more reasonably priced.

You don't need Rosemary Clooney's song to get a clue about the benefits of the pomegranate.

PROPOLIS: IT MAY *BEE* VERY HELPFUL FOR PAIN AND BACTERIA

Recently, my sister experienced dental problems involving tooth and gum pain, headache and possible infection. Amazingly, her dentist, who prefers natural remedies, treated her with bee propolis, rather than antibiotics or pain killers, Lo and behold, within an hour of taking the propolis, her pain subsided. The pain returned the next day and she resolved it once again with the propolis. My sister provided me with a research review on propolis and I was surprised to learn of the healing properties of this substance. Her dentist always suggests patients who have undergone tooth extraction, undergo a prophylactic course of propolis.

What is propolis?

Propolis is a resinous substance collected by worker bees. It is obtained from tree bark, buds, trunk wounds and leaves of various trees and shrubs. Honeybees gather the propolis and mix the resin with nectar (beeswax), which creates a mix of wax, pollen and bee bread. Bees protect their hives by using the propolis to strengthen the actual structure of the hive and to guard it from microbes and fungus. Bees place the propolis at the entrance of the hive where it serves to decontaminate the bees as they enter and exit.

Anti-inflammatory and anti-microbial

The anti-microbial aspect alone explains why this might be useful in human treatment. Bee propolis contains 38 flavonoids and various phenols, which are all strong anti-oxidants. These combinations also create an anti-inflammatory effect. Some of the latest medical research indicates that many diseases begin with an inflammatory process, Propolis has little nutritional value, although it does contains some vitamins and trace minerals. It is used mostly for its anti-fungal, anesthetic and antibiotic qualities. Propolis as a natural antibiotic/anti fungal is even older than the Greek father of medicine, Hippocrates, of whom it is written, prescribed it for promotion of healing wounds and ulcers. This ancient healing substance fell out of fashion years ago, but is now making a come back and is being studied aggressively in several countries.

Clinical studies have found propolis to be helpful internally for many conditions from bronchitis and influenza to external use for ringworm and various skin fungi. As in my sister's case, it is also being used effectively for dental disorders involving pain, infection and inflammation.

One American study found it to be useful for hip joint disease caused by aseptic necrosis of the thigh bone. While 22 patients were treated with aqueous injections of propolis, 32 were treated with routine methods. The most significant improvements occurred in the group using the propolis.

Various other studies have shown propolis to promote tissue repair. Bulgarian studies have found that it inhibits the bacterium that creates stomach ulcers (h-pylori) as well as infections such as the dreaded MRSA, (a staph infection mostly found/contracted in hospitals). An additional study found propolis to be synergistic when combined with antibiotic therapy in treatment of some staph infections. Recent Japanese research has found that propolis activates immune cells which Japanese researchers believe may be helpful in treatment of cancerous tumors. Japan is one of those countries aggressively researching propolis.

Anesthetic effects

Propolis and some of its components were found to produce an anesthetic effect, when tested in rabbits. The anesthetic effect has been shown to be produced by pinocembrin, pinostrobin, and caffeic acid, all components of propolis. A 1996 study found that propolis had effects similar to that of Indomethacin, when used as an anti-inflammatory.

Not for everyone

As with any substance on earth, natural or chemical, propolis is not for everyone. Those who are allergic to bee venom should be very careful and must be under a physician's care before considering its use. Contact dermatitis has been reported in a very few cases by beekeepers, however, once daily contact with the raw product was ceased, the dermatitis immediately resolved. If dermatitis occurs while using propolis, it is recommended that its use be stopped.

Propolis is gaining new respect, not only because of the latest studies, but because advances in science have allowed researchers to test individual components of the substance for targeted responses on specific diseases.

Honey bees pollinate our food supply and provide us with healing substances. Their population has decreased in the U.S. due to insecticide use. Bumbles bees, the large fuzzy bees we see flitting from flower to flower are also very helpful to us.

As for those annoying yellow jackets that hang around our picnic food, they are wasps and can be quite dangerous which I discovered when they attacked my son after building a nest in our attic. They found their way into his bed and when he rolled over, disturbing them, they attacked. They have no use I know of and professional exterminators should be called if they build nests around your property.

PROSTATE—DOES VITAMIN D PLAY A ROLE?

Sometimes the medical community completely ignores what would otherwise be an astonishing revelation. Such is the case as reported by Dr. Jay Rowen *Second Opinion* in his February 2005 newsletter. Rowen discusses two articles published last year. One was in the *New England Journal of Medicine* (NEJM), the other appeared in *Urology*.

Amazingly, an article written by the original advocate of the (prostate-specific antigen) PSA test for prostate cancer, Dr. Thomas Stanley, actually reversed his first clarion call for global PSA testing. It seems in a large study, the PSA test was not as accurate as once believed. Dr. Stanley discussed the study that was exceptionally disappointing when using PSA testing for detecting prostate cancer in men. Dr. Stanley stated, "The PSA era is over in the United States." He then goes on to say, "Our study raises a very serious question of whether a man should even use the PSA for prostate cancer screening anymore…." The article explains that additionally, Dr. Stanley does not believe prostate removal is always the answer to treating prostate cancer. Dr. Rowen paraphrases the report and goes so far as to say that regular PSA levels are not accurate detectors unless the levels are "above 15."

Rowen suggests that if a PSA test is to be relied upon to any degree, the test to be taken is known as "free PSA" which is a more accurate detector of prostate cancer. The higher your "free" PSA, the lower your risk for cancer, according to Rowen.

So what's a man to do?

Plenty, according to Rowen. He states, "If you want to prevent prostate cancer, I strongly urge you have your vitamin D levels checked regularly." Rowen says adequate vitamin D levels are essential to prostate health. Correcting vitamin D deficiencies will reduce your risk of cancer by 80 percent, according to the doctor.

Rowen points out that medical experts are calling for a revision in the required daily dosage of vitamin D which he states can be as high as 10,000 international units (IU's) without becoming toxic. Rowen routinely measures vitamin D as "25-hydroxyvitamin D." He states the ideal levels should be at 45-50 ng/ml or 115-128 nmol/l. He believes most men and women do not reach those levels. Rowen explains, "I currently have almost all of my male patients on a D3 supplement or cod liver oil (4,000 IU daily." He also suggests that men have "common sense" exposure to sunlight.

In researching additional information about prevention of prostate cancer, I found research on saw palmetto, beta sitosterol, pygeum, pumpkin seed extract and vitamin E. These supplements appear to be useful in attaining prostate health. Additionally, I've read that ground flaxseed is also helpful while flaxseed oil alone is not.

In the March 2, 2005 issue of the *Journal of the National Cancer Institute*, a study was released showing vitamin E can reduce prostate cancer risk by 32 percent. As I've written of in the past, according to Dr. Joseph Mercola, the most balanced form of vitamin E is in the form of mixed tocopherols and should always contain "gamma" as well as "alpha" tocopherols. Mercola also points out that seven of 10 men diagnosed with prostate cancer will die from other causes than the prostate cancer.

Dr. Mercola also always reminds patients that diet is the major factor in prevention of all disease.

One of the interesting common threads in so many of these health reports is that a deficiency of one or more vital nutrients can throw the body off kilter and lead to numerous diseases.

Most alternative physicians recommend avoiding sugars, fats and dairy products. Other recommended helps for the prostate and overall general health are green tea, garlic, citrus pectin, quercetin, L-glutamine and N-acetyl-cysteine. Many of these are contained in some ready-made prostate preparations.

When deciding on a prostate formula, read the label and make certain a reputable company with standardized ingredients produces the product. It would be wise for you to write the ingredients on a sheet of paper and give them to your physician to insure he or she knows what you are taking. That same advice applies to all herbs and vitamins. Your physician should always be aware of any supplements you are taking.

RELAXING: VARIOUS ALTERNATIVE VIEWS TO EASE STRESS LEVELS HIBISCUS AND RELORA

We are living in uncertain and tumultuous times, and even if we don't outwardly realize it, we are processing world issues. Sometimes the stress affects us without our being aware of it. Stress manifests itself in higher blood pressure, anxiety and various seemingly unrelated discomforts, all transpiring while we may believe we are coping well.

In this high-tech age, Americans have developed some bad habits. One of the nasty habits we have developed is that we watch television news shows during the dinner hour. Another bad habit is that we watch TV news before going to bed. I have done both. I'm a regular news junkie, but I am in the process of trying to break the habit. Watching TV news during our dinner hour can be disruptive to the digestive process. When we watch the news prior to going to bed, it can interfere with our ability to sleep. Now that war is in the news, it's even more difficult.

Relax with Hibiscus tea

Hibiscus tea is a favorite in the Middle-East, Caribbean and Mexico as well as much of Europe. The hibiscus flowers from the hibiscus sabdariffa (also known as roselle or Jamaica sorrell), family provide much more than mere visual delight. (Most of what we see in the U.S. in the form of hibiscus are cultivars and not very suitable for the teas). Hibiscus tea in many countries is as common as coffee is in the United States. It is said that hibiscus tea is as old as the Pharaohs.

Hibiscus tea, made with the petals of the hibiscus provide several benefits, among them, according to Dr. David Williams, a biochemist, and author of "Alternatives" newsletter, is a reduction in blood pressure. Williams refers to a study, in which participants drank 3 cups of hibiscus sabdariffa tea per day. After 12 days, blood pressure was reduced 11.7% systolic (top number) and 10.4% diastolic (bottom number).

For that occasional mild anxiety, another most promising relaxant is another flower by the name of magnolia officinalis that is used in traditional Chinese medicine. Magnolia bark contains essential oils, alkaloids and biphenols. It is the biphenols, especially "honokiol" that are believed to be the active ingredient that helps give anti-anxiety properties to the magnolia and studies have shown that when it was compared to Valium, it had the same type of calming effects, yet it did not interfere with motor skills or cause drowsiness. A footnote was that Valium created more muscle relaxation than the magnolia; however, the research showed that there were no withdrawal symptoms among patients after stopping magnolia. A product that contains the magnolia bark along with Phellodrendron amurense, another traditional Chinese herb used for relaxation, is known as Relora. Relora is said to be good for occasional mild anxiety and can be found at health food stores.

Another of my favorites for relaxing is to have a massage. As far as I'm concerned, massage is the most relaxing and therapeutic treatment around. If you've never had a professional massage, you are truly missing something that will rejuvenate your entire system.

I searched many pharmaceutical web sites to gather information on the medications available for both sleep disturbances and anxiety. You wouldn't believe the number. Just looking at the sales figures, it is apparent that stress is epidemic and pharmaceutical stocks may well be the safest investment. The problem is, that many prescription and non-prescription drugs create side effects such as dizziness, foggy thinking (a state I can attain without drugs) and grogginess. I thought it would be interesting to see what natural remedies are recommended within the alternative health community for both anxiety and sleep problems.

The amino acid, tryptophan and the hormone melatonin have been utilized with limited success for many people. Melatonin is a hormone produced by the pineal gland in response to darkness. It is believed that melatonin may not be very helpful to those suffering chronic fatigue syndrome (CFS) because some patients with chronic fatigue actually possess an over-abundance of melatonin that can create that tired feeling, even during the day. More studies will have to be conducted to establish this link.

Relaxing with L-theanine

I've gathered exciting research on another amino acid responsible for indirectly creating a more relaxed state. The amino acid is L-theanine, which is found abundantly in green tea and certain mushrooms. L-theanine is unique in that it is helpful in creating a relaxed state without putting one in la-la land. Hence, L-theanine promotes a better sleep environment. We can drink green tea, which contains caffeine, without having the jitters, because L-theanine is a caffeine antagonist. It counteracts the caffeine effect.

The process by which L-theanine can help us relax is that it appears to play a role in allowing the formation of the brain chemical, Gamma Amino Butyric Acid (GABA), which is responsible for both relaxation and giving us that sense of "well being." Studies indicate it actually enhances the thinking process. A Reuters Health article reported on studies conducted at the University of Utah School of Medicine, in Salt Lake City, in which GABA was shown to stop the aging process in the brains of older monkeys.

Another observation of the promise of L-theanine is in noting that Japan has already recognized its usefulness and has approved its use in many food products. Japan is a country with one of the most overworked and over-stressed populations. According to author Bill Faloon of Life Extension Foundation, the Japanese government has approved theanine for addition to many foods and beverages.

In 2003, Science Magazine reported that GABA inducing drugs (such as the amino acid L-theanine) appear to be part of a newer discovery in helping to preserve brain function in the elderly as well as creating a chemical balance that promotes better mental function. L-theanine can be purchased in a form isolated from green tea to provide more directed benefits. The most positive aspect of the research findings is that it appears to have no side effects. For those who have stress and anxiety problems as well as sleep disorders, L-theanine research holds great promise in promoting a healthy sleep pattern, while helping to balance brain chemistry.

SAMBUCOL: KILLS FLU VIRUS

During the harsh 1992-1993 Israeli B/Panama influenza outbreak, virologist, Dr. Madeleine Mumcuoglu, was afforded the opportunity of conducting a small clinical trial to test her research on flu patients. While the test was a small one, the results clearly showed her research to be very successful.

Dr. Mumcuoglu, an Israeli scientist, studying immunology and hematology, began her trials with two groups. The first group was given four tablespoons per day of an "extract." The second group was given a placebo. Within 24 hours, 20% of the group taking the "extract" showed a dramatic reduction in their flu symptoms. After the second day, 75% of those taking her "extract" showed improvement; by the third day 90% had totally recovered. In the untreated placebo group, only 8% showed improvement after 24 hours; the other 92% of those patients showed no improvement until after six days.

Black Elderberry kills viruses?

What was most amazing was that Dr. Mumcuoglu prepared the "extract" from the Black Elderberry (Sambucus Nigra) plant! She was able to isolate the active constituents in the Elderberry that made it effective against virus invasion.

A virus cannot replicate by itself. A virus contains spikes that pierce host cell outer membranes. They also contain an enzyme (neuraminidase) which helps dissolve the cell walls. Dr. Mumcuoglu discovered that constituents in black elderberry bind the spikes, thus disabling them. The high concentrations of bioflavonoids in elderberry help neutralize the action of viral spike enzymes at the same time. Her supervisor, Dr. Jean Lindeman, of interferon fame, encouraged Dr. Mumcuoglu's study of the Black Elderberry. She then developed a food product known as Sambucol, made from the black elderberry.

Scientific Studies

There are eight scientific publications with positive results on the study of black elderberry and its anti-viral properties.

In other studies, Sambucol was found to have inhibited several other strains of virus by strengthening cell membranes.

The European Cytokine Network (Vol. 12, Issue 2, June 2001) published a research paper showing Sambucol enhances the immune system and increases the production of white blood cell cytokines (proteins produced primarily by white blood cells that regulate immune reaction). Additionally, a Kimron Veterinary Institute study in Israel found that Sambucol neutralized the West Nile virus in animals. It makes sense since elderberry, has broad-spectrum anti-viral properties. Most all berries, in general, are high in antioxidants. Blueberries deliciously included.

I first heard of the product through medical newsletters about five years ago. Dr. David Williams and Dr. Andrew Weil have spoken highly of Sambucol so I decided that since it was neither a chemical nor a dangerous herb, I would try it. Considering I cannot take most pharmaceuticals, it is necessary for me to research alternative methods for most everything. I can honestly say it has performed well for my family and numerous others who noted my use of it. I take it at the first sign of flu and so far, for the last five years, it has proven effective.

SAM-E: TRIPLE BENEFITS FOR DEPRESSION, OSTEOARTHRITIS AND LIVER HEALTH

A naturally occurring compound found in every cell in the human body has shown promise for what would seem three unrelated conditions. The compound is known as SAMe (S-Adenosyl-L-methionine) and has been shown in clinical trials to be helpful with depression, osteoarthritis as well as being helpful in promoting liver health. While it is useful for depression, it is not helpful for those with bipolar disorders (manic depression).

NOTE: It is suggested that people with bipolar disorders avoid using SAMe.

A U.S. government Evidence Report/Technology Assessment: Number 64 entitled "S-Adenosyl-L-Methionine for Treatment of Depression, Osteoarthritis and Liver Disease" is a collection of data from numerous published studies conducted around the world in the year 2000.

The government accepted 47 studies on Depression, 14 on Osteoarthritis and 41 on liver disease. The study concluded that larger and longer trials are in order to more conclusively confirm the promising results of the initial assessment.

The studies on depression showed that there was not a significant difference between the conventional pharmacologic medications prescribed for depression and SAMe. In other words, SAMe performed as well as the medications in relieving depression. The cost was appreciably lower for SAMe when compared to prescription medications.

How does SAMe work for depression?

According to an article appearing in *Life Extension (LE) Magazine*, (January 2005), SAMe is believed to increase the synthesis of "neurotransmitters that are crucial to normal mood, behavior and emotion." Interestingly, the article explains, "Although normally abundant, SAMe levels decline with age and drop dramatically during bouts of depression." The author further reports, "A noticeable drop in SAMe levels is also associated with neurological disorders such as Alzheimer's disease, Parkinson's disease and dementia due to HIV complications" according to reports cited in LE. SAMe is "assembled" from two building blocks: an amino acid, methionine, and adenosine triphosphate (ATP) an energy component. When working together, they allow the brain to manufacture dopamine, serotonin and norepinephrine.

In order to work effectively, SAMe needs the help of methionine." Adequate levels of methionine depend on the availability of folic acid and vitamin B12. "Depression has been associated with a deficiency in either of these vitamins," according to a clinical study cited in the article.

The article quotes Richard Brown, M.D., assistant professor of clinical psychiatry at Colombia University as stating patients feel better and energized within days of starting. He states he even uses it for children with attention deficit disorder.

How does SAMe work for osteoarthritis

It may "reverse the cartilage degeneration that triggers inflammation in the first place," according to the LE article. The article further explains that a report published in the British Journal of Rheumatology "concluded that SAMe reversed various indicators of joint tissue damage elicited in the laboratory by tumor necrosis factor-alpha, a dangerous cytokine implicated in a variety of inflammatory diseases."

All studies explain that it is important not to discontinue taking present medications.

Yet other reports cited in the article state that SAMe increases proteoglycan synthesis and proliferation rate, thus providing chondroprotective effects." In other words, it attracts and holds water necessary for cartilage function in the joints.

How does it work for the liver?

Once again, SAMe was shown to facilitate more than 100 different reaction that not only help the brain and joints, but the liver. It promotes the production of glutathione within the body. Glutathione is known as a tremendous antioxidant that assists the liver in attaching to toxins and making them water soluble, hence, allowing them to be flushed from the body.

The article further explains, "Because SAMe is so important to the liver, up to 80% of methionine in the liver is converted to SAMe. Oral SAMe has been shown to increase glutathione levels in the liver and red blood cells" once again, according to studies cited in LE magazine.

If you intend to seek information about SAMe for depression, it's essential that you speak with your physician about making the change. The article warns patients not to stop taking present medications, but to have their physicians seek further information about SAMe.

SEASONAL AFFECTIVE DISORDER (SAD)

There can be numerous causes for mild depression and the winter blahs. One of the most common causes is a condition known as Seasonal Affective Disorder (SAD). During the winter months, there seems to be a lack of bright light. The days are shorter and darker and snow clouds can hang out for lengthy periods, making the darkness even more apparent. For some people who are especially sensitive to this lack of bright light, these changes can result in a case of feeling down in the dumps.

Among the speculations as to why this disorder exists is the theory that the pineal gland which produces a sleep hormone known as melatonin, may not get enough light to fully awaken us during daytime hours, and serotonin, a neurotransmitter in the brain that helps us to fight depression, may also not be adequately produced.

Signs of SAD

Fatigue, feeling blue, sleep problems, lethargy, and overeating are among the problems associated with SAD. Some people actually experience joint pain and stomach problems during this period of time. Younger children may even display behavioral disorders

Why do only some people become affected?

That is a mystery. It's also about brain chemistry and the causes are still partly unknown, but it is known that the pineal gland which produces a sleep hormone known as Melatonin, may not get enough light to fully awaken us during the day, and serotonin, a neurotransmitter in the brain that helps us to fight depression, may also not be adequately produced.

Lights to the rescue

Studies have shown that bright lights increased production of serotonin during these months. The sight of snow actually helps, probably because snow makes everything bright and white. There are actually "light boxes" you can purchase for use during the winter months if you feel that lack of light may be part of the cause of your blues.

Happy fats and brain food

Cardiologist, Stephen Sinatra, has a few suggestions for those who are facing mild depression from SAD or any other cause during the winter months, but his suggestions can be helpful all year round.

He recommends foods that help your brain release endorphins. Foods that feed your brain. The most recent findings are that a balance between omega-6 and omega-3 fats is part of the key to healthy brain function. The healthy fats we need come from fish oils, nuts, seed, ground flaxseed, DHA-fortified eggs (purchased in health food stores), complex carbohydrates that are found in fruits and vegetables and whole grains; particularly, things like brown rice, wild rice and barley. He also recommends organic turkey, avocados and honey. Again, he recommends a modified Mediterranean diet, which includes extra virgin olive oil instead of butter or margarines, more vegetables and less red meat.

The foods he suggests (along with our supplements) contain essential fatty acids that feed the entire body, especially the brain. These fatty acids trigger chemical reactions that cause our brains and bodies to produce other chemicals that assist in sustaining our general health.

He says it's important that we do not confuse unhealthy hydrogenated and saturated fats such as those in French fries and other fried foods and margarines, with the good fats contained in extra virgin olive oil, seeds, nuts and fish oils. The unhealthy fats actually work against us and reverse good mental and physical health.

Exercise also produces what are known as the most effective endorphins; beta-endorphins according to Dr. Sinatra. So between, proper light, diet and exercise, we can help fight the winter blahs while maintaining better mental and physical health. Supplements may interfere with your other medications. Your physician should be aware of any vitamins, herbs or minerals you are taking.

SHINGLES—VARIOUS VIEWS AND TREATMENTS

It may begin with a tingling or numbing sensation; itching or unexplained pain that mimics muscle aches. A blister type chicken pox-type rash will appear in a few days. The pain may become severe and travel along nerve paths. We're talking shingles (varicella zoster/herpes zoster). Shingles affect only one side of the body and most typically appears along the waistline, however, it can show up anywhere including on the face in which case, medical help should be sought to avoid eye involvement.

Anyone who has had chicken pox or the chicken pox vaccination can suffer from shingles decades later. The chicken pox virus remains within nerve cells near the spinal cord to become an opportunist disease, reactivating when the immune system is compromised. Emotional stress, other non-related diseases and skin trauma or even sunburn can reactivate the virus. Shingles is most common among those over age 50 but mostly strikes the elderly. The outbreak can be negligible or so painful it can require hospitalization. It can result in a secondary disorder known as post-herpetic neuralgia, a painful recurring disorder of the nerve fibers that may last for months at a time. The key appears to lie in prompt treatment at the first signs of an outbreak.

I have searched numerous sites for information from both conventional and alternative sources regarding causes and treatment of the disorder. Among the informative resources are the National Institute of Neurological Disorders and Stroke as well as alternative physician, Joseph Mercola, D.O.

A May 2002, article printed in the *Journal of the American Medical Association* (JAMA), published a study by British public health scientists that concluded the mandatory chicken pox vaccination might pose problems in the future. A mathematical model predicted that while the chicken pox vaccine may eliminate the generally mild childhood disease in the United States, it could very well result in 21 million additional cases of the more serious disorder, shingles. This gives credence to the argument that sometimes the cure is worse than the disease. The British scientists believe that adults, who are exposed to children with childhood chicken pox, actually benefit because the exposure acts as a booster vaccine, inhibiting the reactivation of shingles.

Conventional Treatment—The main treatment for shingles consists of antiviral medication: Zovirax, Famvir, and Valtrex. Other conventional treatment can include tricyclic anti-depressants. They are believed to work on certain neurotransmitters that send out pain signals. For severe cases a machine known as transcutaneous electrical nerve stimulation TENS) is employed. The machine sends small electrical impulses to the electrodes that are placed along the painful body regions. The TENS unit then sends impulses to the nerves in the skin. Lidoderm Cream/Lidoderm Patch (5 percent Lidocaine) is another form of treat-

ment for the pain. Another Food and Drug Administration (FDA) approved topical cream is Capsaicin (cayenne). It works for some and is caustic to others.

Alternative Treatment—Alternative physicians believe that by taking proteolytic
(protein digesting) enzymes in the early stages of shingles, an outbreak can be
milder or even entirely abated. Proteolytic enzymes facilitate the digestion of protein. They include papain (from papaya), bromelain (from pineapple), trypsin
and chymotrypsin taken from animal sources. In a double-blind study of 190
active shingles patients, proteolytic enzymes were compared against acyclovir.
Both groups experienced similar pain relief, but the enzyme-treated group
showed fewer side effects. Proteolytic enzymes provide other health benefits as
well, while conventional antivirals, can pose serious side effects.

In one study, the application of honey was also tried against acyclovir with 43
percent better results than the acyclovir, according to Dr. Jonathan Wright. He
also reminds his readers to avoid peanuts, beans, seeds and grains as well as other
foods that are high in L-arginine. Sugar and foods that create allergic reactions are
also culprits in herpes outbreaks, according to Dr. Wright. He suggests supplementation with vitamin C, selenium and lithium because they inhibit herpes
reproduction. He suggests 15-20 mg. of lithium and 400 to 500 mcg of selenium
per day while treating the herpes outbreak.

Many alternative physicians to relieve the itching and pain use natural topical
anti-viral products such as "Shingles No More" and Herp-Eeze. Apple cider vinegar is an age-old remedy used for itching. My mom soaked cloths with apple
cider and applied them directly to the skin. The chicken pox seemed to dry up
quickly. A few cups in the bathwater became part of her treatment for relief from
the itching of all kinds. The amino acid L-lysine and vitamin B1 (thiamine)
appear to provide some degree of effectiveness against all types of herpes, including cold sores, according to Wright.

"Shingles No More" can be purchased at 323-296-7770, and Herpes-eeze:
The Next Generation can be purchased at 800-753-1981. HPX and HPX2 can
be obtained through Dr. Wright's Tahoma Clinic. Call 425-264-0059.

SINUS/FUNGUS CONNECTION?

We all have at least one friend or family member who suffers from a condition
known as chronic sinusitis. Chronic sinusitis can become debilitating in some
people and disrupt their daily living activities. Their ability to think past the pain

and discomfort can caused them to suffer depression in addition to the chronic sinusitis. Many doctors have treated sinusitis with a course of antibiotics. In some cases, antibiotics have actually exacerbated the symptoms. Unless there is a bacterial component clearly present, studies have shown that antibiotics are not effective for the treatment of sinus congestion or sinusitis.

There is no doubt that sinusitis can create as much discomfort as any painful disease on the planet, yet, "old habits die hard," and ineffective treatments continue to prevail, even considering new research that can explain why antibiotics have been the least effective approach in treating the condition.

The key may have begun to take form in a Mayo Clinic study that found most cases of chronic sinusitis are due to fungus infections, not bacterial growth. According to the study, the discomfort associated with these fungus infections, is merely the body's immune system response to the fungus. This fungus connection explains why antibiotics have not been as successful in treatment of sinusitis. Antibiotics kill bacteria not fungi. Antibiotics can, in fact, facilitate the growth of yeast. They do this by destroying our "friendly bacteria" which is essential to our immune system function, allowing the fungus to move in and proliferate. This kill-off of necessary critters, creates a chain reaction in the body that results in making our bodies even less capable of dealing with other harmful invading organisms and can cause severe yeast growth.

Television nutritionist, Doug Kaufman, has authored a book "*The Fungus Link*" in which he posits a fungus connection is associated with sinus problems and many other common diseases, including some forms of depression.

Kaufman's fungus theory is supported by the Mayo Clinic research, but he takes it to another level, postulating that fungus growth is the basis of many diseases. He believes our lifestyles, antibiotic and hormone treated cattle, added to the liberal use of antibiotics in the U.S. has created little villages of fungus growth, that interfere with our immune function.

The fungus theory may be something to examine more closely considering the results of another study involving children with sinus problems.

Joseph Mercola, D.O. a Schaumburg alternative physician, says studies have shown that children with cough, runny nose and sinus problems are unlikely to respond to antibiotics. He sites a study in which children with acute sinusitis for 10 days or longer were given either an inactive placebo pill or antibiotics. The study showed the placebo group was just as likely to recover as children prescribed antibiotics. Mercola says, "Symptoms improved within 7 days in 81% of children in each group and within 10 days in 87% of all children." The study was conducted using Amoxicillin or Augmentin as the antibiotic.

Treatment for fungus

Among the various treatments for fungus, Doug Kaufman, suggests Diflucan and Nystatin, which are pharmaceutical drugs used to treat yeast infections. These pharmaceuticals must be prescribed by a physician. (Some alternative doctors are not comfortable using either Diflucan or Nystatin and recommend more natural products which may take longer to work). Kaufman also feels we must supplement with acidophilus, the "friendly bacteria" our intestines need. He believes that changing diet habits is just as important as killing off the excess fungus. He believes the elimination of dairy products and eliminating gluten containing foods, will help the body fight the thickened mucous in nasal passages. He is also one of those who feel refined sugars; sodas and sweets must be eliminated as well. He suggests a diet that boosts the immune system.

Dr. Mercola also feels that sinusitis could be fungus, allergic and even viral in nature.

Various suggestions by alternative physicians

1. Using a saline nasal spray on a daily basis would help prevent sinusitis attacks. It is said to cleanse the area and keep the mucous thin to prevent the build-up of fungus and bacteria. I have seen this work for some of my own family members.
2. Avoid dairy foods and wheat

Perhaps, eliminating dairy and gluten products will do the trick. You may want to try the nasal spray in combination with a change in diet. It's a good idea to search the alternative web sites and look at some of the other recommendations that might fit your particular situation. We are all individuals and what is good for one may not be good for another. For that reason, try what works best for you. Some times it takes a little time, but it will be worth the effort. Below are some of the products recommended.

Product #1

For a number of years, I have read the praises of a nasal spray known as Xlear (pronounced "clear,") Nasal Wash by Dr. David Williams, a biochemist and researcher. Williams explains that the product has many uses in both adults and children because it contains Xylitol, another of the sugar fractions and a substitute for table sugar. Xylitol is frequently found in chewing gums and toothpaste and is used by diabetics for sweetening. It is derived from birch trees, cane, corn cobs and corn stalks.

The nasal spray, Xlear, contains xylitol, purified water, saline and grape seed extract. Grape seed is a strong anti-oxidant. According to Dr. Williams, reports have shown xylitol to be a natural enemy of bacteria. While xylitol is not an antibiotic, it inhibits bacteria such as strep, pneumo and H flu from adhering to nasal mucous membrane, exactly in the same fashion as d-mannose (another healthful sugar fraction) in cranberry juice, inhibits bacteria from "sticking" to the walls of the bladder. Xlear Nasal Spray flushes and hydrates nasal passages. Xylitol in gum also possesses dental benefits, in that it prevents tooth decay; again, by precluding the streptococcus mutans, a bacteria that causes decay, from adhering to teeth or local membrane in the mouth. Once the concept of xylitol's ability to inhibit bacteria adherence is understood, it will most likely have wider application, especially since studies have been promising in showing its ability to reduce the occurrence of acute otitis media (ear infections).

Dr. Williams suggests the nasal passages should be flushed on a regular basis. The fact that it is not an antibiotic makes it safer to use regularly. Dr. Williams suggests that we make certain to use it daily during flu season.

Product #2

Dr. Williams also discovered a German product containing five herbs that work synergistically to enhance the body's inflammatory process as well as mucus production. None of the herbs work alone but combined they assist in promoting sinus health, according to Williams. He states it will help keep the sinuses drained in most cases. The herbs are Common Sorrell, Cowslip (flower) European Elder (flower), European Vervain (herb) and Gentian (root). The product is used pharmaceutically in Germany and undergoes strict German government standards.

It can be purchased by going to drdavidwilliams.com. Fifty tablets are $12.99.

The Centers for Disease Control and Prevention have established that washing hands helps to eliminate passing along bacteria; however, most bacteria gain entrance through nasal passages, so attention to the sinus area appears to be very essential in fighting sinus maladies.

Product #3

According to the folks at Health Science Institute, another product working on a separate concept for hay fever and other allergy sufferers, is Sneeze-eze. It was developed for allergy and hay fever sufferers in the United Kingdom under the name Nasaleze. It's a simple vegetable powder with no pharmacologic action; yet, when it is introduced into the nasal passages it creates a mucous protection. The very concept of the product is that not enough healthy mucous is available to filter pollutants and allergens from the nasal passages and that the product will serve to create enough healthy mucous to effectively filter allergens.

In 2003, a study on hay fever sufferers was conducted using Nasaleze (Sneeze-eze) common allergy prescription and non-prescription medications on the market today as well as a placebo group. Pollen measurements were taken on a daily basis during the period of the test. The findings will appear in the September 2003, issue of "Alternatives in Natural Therapy." The results indicated that the hay fever sufferers in the study found Nasaleze (Sneeze-eze) much more effective than the prescription medications they were using for allergies. A most positive side-effect of using the product was that concurrently during the study, several sufferers with hay fever who also suffered mild atopic dermatitis, found that their atopic dermatitis had cleared. Next spring, studies will be conducted in the United Kingdom using Nasaleze (Sneeze-eze) for mild atopic dermatitis. If you suffer mild atopic dermatitis, you may wish to participate in the trials. This is only for cases of atopic and not stress related dermatitis.

Product #4

Another great nasal spray is the German made Sinupret. It is especially useful for inflammation of the paranasal passages It is made from primrose flowers, gentian root, elder flowers, common sorrel herb and shop vervain wort. Sinupret enhances antibiotic therapy and also acts as an antiviral according to the makers. It keeps the nasal passages clear if used on a regular basis. It is top drawer according to Dr. Jonathn Wright.

The important thing to consider when using alternative methods for any disorder is that the results may not be as instantaneous as with prescribed medications. It's essential to hang in there and give nature a chance to heal. Temporarily masking symptoms is not healing. The present condition of your nasal passages will also have an effect in how quickly it may work. In the study, relief was obtained in as little as 10 minutes among those with recent onset of hay fever.

If you cannot find the products at your local health food store, you can call: (Xlear) 1-877-599-5327 (Sneeze-eze) 1-800-247-5731. I would like feedback from those using the products on the effectiveness of the products.

STATIN DRUG WARNINGS: CRESTOR, VYTORIN

Also see (coenzyme Q10—Heart and Cellular Energy)

The Consumer Watchdog Group, Public Citizen, has requested that the Food & Drug Administration (FDA) immediately remove one of the newest statin drugs from the market. That drug is Crestor and according to Public Citizen, an analysis of adverse drug reaction reports found "the rate of reports of kidney failure or damage among patients taking Crestor is 75 times higher than in all patients taking all other statin drugs." They also reported that the new analysis also found muscle breakdown in patients taking Crestor was approaching that of Baycol (cervistatin), a drug that was recalled several years ago.

Additionally, the publication warns about problems with two new drugs for the treatment of cholesterol. The newer drugs are Zetia (Ezetimibe) and Vytorin (Ezetimibe with simivastatin). They recommend that especially older patients not use these drugs until the year 2009. The reason for this delay is that true side effects are often observed only after new drugs have been widely used for a few years. In other words, many people are akin to guinea pigs when using new drugs.

The problems they list with the new cholesterol drugs are that clinical trials showed even higher incidence of elevated blood enzyme creatinine phosphokinase (CPK). This enzyme indicates muscle toxicity which can be fatal. In addition to the above conditions, reports of hypersensitivity reactions, angioedema (serious and dangerous swelling), inflammation of the gallbladder, gallstones, pancreatitis and nausea were also among complaints to the FDA with the newer drugs.

One of the suggestions for physicians whose patients have elevated LDL cholesterol and other elevated blood fats was to first screen the patient for various conditions such as diabetes, hypothyroidism (low thyroid), chronic kidney failure or the use of progestins, steroids and corticosteroids, which raise LDL levels.

Many of these drugs may be useful in certain cases when absolutely necessary. The key is in determining through the process of eliminating other disorders as a cause of the symptoms and changing something as simple as diet. Always remember, when a new drug makes it to the market, the only way the company developing the drug can recover costs is by encouraging widespread use of that drug. Think about it. That isn't always good for patients.

SKIN CARE AND SUNSCREEN

Evergreen Park, Illinois is fortunate to have young pediatrician, Dr. Van Koinis caring for area children. I guess we might refer to Dr. Koinis as an integrative physician because he has an innate ability to know when to use conventional medicine and when natural is better.

One of his most immediate areas of concern is exposure of young skin to the elements, especially ultra violet radiation.

Don't rely on sun screen

"Most patients are unaware that sunscreens provide little protection from UVA, the sun's longer rays. These are the rays that cause melanomas" says Dr. Koinis. Among his problems with sunscreens are 1) they contain chemicals, 2) the ingredients are not standardized, and 3) the advertising implies they provide full protection when they do not. "Sunscreens are actually prepared for the shorter UVB rays and even at that, sunscreen must be aggressively re-applied to provide just a moderate amount of protection," he said. He points out that the aging process from sun damage takes place even with sunscreens. His concern is that while sunscreen application is better than nothing at all, people must be aware that it is only of limited assistance in protecting skin. Most of us have always felt that as long as we apply sunscreen we can safely bask in the sun. That is a dangerous assumption and he hopes to disabuse us of that dangerous concept. Dr. Koinis states we must protect our skin all 12 months of the year, not just in summer.

He shows the parents of his patients how to prepare home remedies containing plentiful, natural ingredients to protect their skin.

A larger concern

Dr. Koinis states that because the skin is the largest organ of the body and difficult to protect, it takes a very healthy immune system to effectively respond to daily stressors such as UV rays and environmental pollutants.

A strong immune system is essential to overall health that includes skin health. He is deeply concerned with the eating habits of the young and feels that proper diet and supplementation are essential to the development of a healthy immune response. Fast food advertising troubles him as well as the soda and fat consumption of our youth.

Dr. Koinis began his search for more natural solutions after becoming frustrated with the pharmaceutical industry and what he considered to be a lack of effectiveness and the serious side-effects of so many chemical skin preparations. He sees the need to address the underlying condition and not just treat the symptoms.

As promised, here are some suggestions of proven natural substances to help build immunity and provide photo protective help as well. They may be purchased at your local store or health food store.

Prevention of sunburn and UV damage: Drink green tea, black tea, lemon tea, (apply it topically too). Eat artichokes and ginger. Dr. Koinis also says Red Clover tea protects from inflammation and immune suppression induced by UV radiation.—Look for the product "EQOL" in any body lotions. They are immunoprotective, more so than sunscreens.

For Sunburn: Extra virgin olive oil actually mitigates DNA damage to some degree. Apply it immediately after exposure to the sun. (Studies show extra virgin olive oil does not provide protection when applied prior to exposure). After exposure, it acts as a skin rescue and helps skin recovery.

For wound healing: Dr. Koinis recommends honey for wound healing and heat burns. It provides moisture, contains antiseptic properties and is anti-inflammatory. He says honey is very effective on Q-tips for mouth ulcers, cold sores, along with green tea, both internally and externally and curcumin (found in turmeric), which is also anti-inflammatory, photo protective and assists in wound healing.

For eczema Milk thistle extract—mix in water and extra virgin olive oil—or with green tea, black tea or oolong tea extract and water.

For acne: Alpha lipoic Acid—taken orally or applied topically, mixed with water and green tea or with milk thistle.

Dr. Koinis has been impressed by the results of these natural plants and their proven healing powers. For the convenience of his patients, he has used his basic research and prepared a preventive and healing cream that is easy to apply, lasts at least 12 hours and is useful for the entire family. The cream helps with most skin disorders and minor skin irritations, bites, and various minor inflammations. It is especially useful as a photo protective agent when one is going to be exposed to the sun (not for sunbathing). His cream fights the assaults of the environment and UV rays. It is anti-inflammatory, anti-carcinogenic and reaches into the deepest layers of skin, stopping the causes of inflammatory conditions. Dr. Koinis explains that the aging process is mostly photo aging, from the elements and that the ingredients in the cream prevent the skin from breaking down due to inflammatory conditions. As we age, our epidermal layer becomes thinner and we become more susceptible to UV radiation and every other assault on the skin. His cream preserves the skin barrier.

SODA: HOW MUCH SUGAR IS IN A CAN? WHAT ELSE CAN SPELL TROUBLE?

We all know that cigarettes post a warning on the carton advising of health hazards associated with smoking; however, we never read that the drive-thru window and the soda vending machine can also be hazardous to your health. One must be in solitary confinement not to be aware of the dangers of too much fat and sugar in both soda and fast foods. What you shouldn't eat and drink can be as important as what you should eat and drink.

Dr. Benjamin Feingold, a man considered to have been a heretic during the 1960's stated our children were hyperactive because of sugar and food additives. Feingold was way ahead of his time.

Thankfully, there are growing numbers of pediatricians and family practitioners that are expressing concern about fast food and the increase in soda consumption among children. The sugar content in one 12 oz. bottle/can of soda may be between 7 and 10 spoonfuls. Add the caffeine and phosphoric acid which is also listed as a main ingredient and you have a tiger by the tail.

A medical news report in the February 27, 2001 issue of the Washington Post, states: "There's growing concern that even a few cans of soda today can be damaging when they are consumed during the peak bone-building years of childhood and adolescence." The Post report further discloses "A 1996 study published in the Journal of Nutrition by the FDA's Office of Special Nutritionals noted that a pattern of high phosphorus/low calcium consumption, common in the American diet, is not conducive to optimizing peak bone mass in young women."

The Post Article further points to a 1994 Harvard study which followed teenage athletes (girls 14 years of age) with bone fractures, and "found a strong association between cola beverage consumption and bone fractures in 14-year-old girls. The girls who drank cola were about five times more likely to suffer bone fractures than girls who didn't consume soda pop."

Dr. Joseph Mercola notes that animal studies have shown that consistent bone loss was observed with the use of colas among rats. Dr. Mercola also points to Lancet, a British medical journal's report that a team of Harvard researchers claimed a link between soft drinks and childhood obesity. The researchers con-

ducted a 19-month study on two groups of 12-year old students; one group consumed no soda, the other drank soda on a regular basis. On an average, children
who drink soda gain 200 additional empty calories per day.

Parent Power

Mercola also writes of a Wisconsin high school district that implemented a
healthy diet in 1997. He states that the results of changing diet have made a difference in grades, behavior and general well being among the students at the high
school and that the program has now been expanded to include a middle school
in the district.

Some organizations take too strident an approach, accusing the soft drink and
fast food industries of everything from personally poisoning for profit, to being
capitalist pigs looking for the buck. They ask an inept government that produces
$900.00 hammers, to intervene. Government intervention is not the answer. Par-
ent intervention is the answer. It's about supply and demand. If we demanded
better, they would supply better. There's no conspiracy, no capitalist pigdom
here, just the need for those who object to the ingredients in various foods and
drinks, to change their eating and drinking habits. Once sales fall, retailers and
producers of soda and fast food will get the message and produce healthier products. However, until parents take control, we will continue to see reports showing
upwards of 56% of 8 year olds drinking soda on a daily basis. Today is the day for
parents to make a serious decision about their children's future.

SOY: IS IT REALLY ALL THAT GOOD?

Have you noticed the ever-increasing presence of soy products as you walk
through the grocery store? Soy milk, soy candy bars, soy meats, soy veggies, soy
everything. At first glance, one might think this trend is taking us into a new
healthy direction, but the latest research might indicate otherwise.

The soy issue wasn't a difficult one for me. I don't like the taste of soy "anything" except soy sauce on occasion when added while cooking a roast. I did my
level best to add soy products to my diet, but fact is, I hated them and thankfully,
for good reason, according to what many newer studies is showing. According to
Sally Fallon and Dr. May Enig, who wrote an article, "Cinderella's Dark Side,"
soy, is not quite as healthful as claimed over the years.

No question about it, there is a huge battle going on in the alternative and conventional health arena regarding soy, with most alternative physicians coming down against soy.

One of the major concerns about soy is that it may not be good for infants as once believed because it contains phytoestrogens and also blocks the absorption of iodine that is necessary for thyroid function. According to Enig and Fallon, parents are being led to believe that soy is good for infants. Of course, if children have allergies to milk, or formula, it may be the only alternative. Enig and Fallon claim the latest studies indicate soy also inhibits some mineral absorption and blocks useful enzymes.

According to Enig and Fallon, "A study from Cornell University, published in the *Journal of the American College of Nutrition*, 1986, which found that children who develop diabetes mellitus were twice as likely to have been fed soy."

They further list, "A November 1994 warning published in Pediatrics (AAP) in which the Nutrition Committee of the American Academy of Pediatrics advised against the use of soy formulas due to the diabetes risk." According to the authors, "These warnings have been neglected ever since it was reported that the AAP accepted a multi-dollar donation from the Infant Formula Council for their new headquarters building outside Chicago."

Enig and Fallon cited numerous studies regarding the problems with soy, however, it seems that once a fad catches on, it's hard to stem the tide.

In two of the studies cited by Enig and Fallon, from a 1997 study that appeared in "Nutrition and Cancer", found that "phytoestrogens at levels close to probable levels in humans stimulate cellular changes leading to breast cancer; the other found that dietary soy suppressed enzymes protective of breast cancer in mice."

Among the many additional studies they cite, is that soy, while it does have phytoestrogens, does not generally assist in alleviating hot flashes or night sweats experienced by women during menopause.

One of the problems with soy is the form in which soy is consumed. The Japanese consume fermented forms of soy, such as that in tofu, meso, natto and do not use it as a main dish but rather as a side dish and eat less than one gram per day.

Among the studies they quote was a 1998 study published in "Toxicology and Industrial Health," showing phytoestrogens as being potential endocrine disrupters in males.

There were enough studies to indicate that perhaps we should reconsider the soy craze that appears to have taken hold in the United States. We seem to have adopted the theory that if a little is good a lot must be even better. Big mistake. A little soy is one thing, but to inundate every food and every aspect of life with soy products may not be that useful and according to the studies referenced may actually be harmful.

I decided to write about soy when I noticed the increasing numbers of soy products being promoted as if it were a miracle drug. I, too, was under the impression that soy was one of the best products around until several of the doctors I admire most, pointed out the "other side of the story."

There is no call for hysteria about soy, but you have a right to know that there seems to be a downside if you consume too much soy in the wrong form. You must decide for yourself, keeping in mind that soy is big business these days.

STEVIA—A BETTER SUBSTITUTE FOR SUGAR

There's good news for those of us who would like to break that "sweet tooth" habit. Even better news is that it's not only sweet and healthy, but it has no calories. It's called "Stevia," a natural plant from Paraguay, 30 times sweeter than cane sugar but without the damaging effects of sugar or some of the complaints associated with the present artificial sweeteners we use. In Paraguay, where stevia has been used for hundreds of years, they refer to it as "honey leaf." There is a compilation of data in booklet form, written by Daniel Mowrey, Ph.D., a well-known researcher of herbal products. He obtained studies on the substance from around the world. He investigated its use and acceptance from continent to continent. In Paraguay and Brazil, doctors prescribe stevia for treatment of both diabetes and hypoglycemia because of its ability to stabilize blood sugar levels. According to Mowrey, "Paraguayans say that stevia is helpful for hypoglycemia and diabetes because it nourishes the pancreas and thereby helps to restore normal pancreatic function."

According to Dr. Mowrey, two of the main constituents of Stevia leaves (glycosides) are what makes it sweet. He says, "Extracted, they are currently being used as sweetening agents in several countries, including Japan, China, Korea, Taiwan, Israel, Uraguay, Brazil, and Paraguay." He further points out that "In Japan, commercialization of stevia was very rapid, beginning with the ban of artificial sweeteners during the 1960's. In 1970 the Japanese National Institute of Health began importing stevia for investigation, and by 1980 it was being used in hundreds of food products throughout the country." Stevia maintains 40% of the sweetener market in Japan.

It seems the most flavorful stevia is grown in Paraguay. However, it is commercially grown and used in many other countries including the U.S. I've tasted it and have begun to use the product. It has never left that artificial sweetener aftertaste.

Sweet leaf inhibits bacteria

The sweet leaf has also been found to inhibit the growth and reproduction of bacteria and other organisms. Mowrey explains, "Research clearly shows that Streptococcus mutans, Pseudomonas aeruginos, Proteus vulgaris and other microbes do not thrive in the presence of the non-nutritive stevia constituents. This fact, combined with the naturally sweet flavor of the herb, makes it a suitable ingredient for mouth washes and for tooth pastes."

Political hurdles

Stevia powder is available in the U.S. at most health food stores; however, it cannot be sold as a sweetener, according to the FDA. In 1995, the Thomas J. Lipton Co. attempted to petition the FDA to allow Lipton to add stevia to some of their products as a "sweetener", but the FDA denied their request. Even though there have been no studies to show it as being toxic at any level, the FDA continues to prohibit it be labeled as a "sweetener" and allows only the present chemical sweeteners to be approved for use as "sweeteners" in the U.S.

In l993, U.S. Senator, Jon Kyle, (R. Ariz.) may have given us a bit of insight as to the politics involved in the FDA's rejection of stevia. In a letter to former FDA Commissioner, David Kessler, Kyle wrote that "(The FDA action on stevia is) a restraint of trade to benefit the artificial sweetener industry."

Sounds like a game. It's very sweet, but you can't purchase it as a "sweetener."

The greatest concern of the artificial sweetener industry is that stevia might someday be approved for incorporation into food and drink production. That would really hurt the sugar and artificial sweetener industry.

Knowing that stevia has been used safely in Japan for 30 years, only after being investigated for l0 solid years, makes me comfortable in trying it. Considering my own allergic reaction to aspartame/NutraSweet makes stevia especially beneficial for me.

"Better living through chemistry?" Not always.

STROKE: DO NUTRIENT DEFICIENCIES PLAY A ROLE?

Years ago early studies indicated an association between high homocysteine levels and the development of stroke, heart attack and atherosclerosis. Homocysteine is an amino acid produced by the body that can be measured through blood testing. Some have a genetic propensity toward high homocysteine while others have high levels because of poor eating habits.

The Lancet, a British medical journal, reported that linkages between homocysteine levels and stroke were becoming more easily documented. A comprehensive analysis of published data has been able to demonstrate the link. This is important because stroke is the third most common cause of death in developed countries.

The January 26, 2005 edition of the American Medical Association (AMA) Journal indicates folic acid helps women prevent heart attack and reduces blood pressure. Even more encouraging is the news that high homocysteine levels can easily be treated. We don't need prescription drugs (although doctors prescribe them anyway). We need an inexpensive supplement known as folic acid. Folic acid is from the B vitamin family and is found in green leafy vegetables and fresh fruits. The word "folic" is derived from the word "foliage." It can also be obtained as a supplement. In fact, according to Dr. Jonathan Wright, up to 50 percent of folate in green leafy vegetables, breaks down within 48 hours of picking the vegetables. The AMA journal study indicated that food alone did not supply the necessary folate. It's apparent we don't obtain our veggies within 48 hours of being picked. According to many other alternative physicians, folic acid should be taken along with B6 and B12 to enhance its absorption abilities.

For years we have been told that the heart health story lies in a simple cholesterol test. While cholesterol may be somewhat of a factor, is it losing ground as the major factor in predicting heart disease, especially since, 50 percent of heart attacks occur among people with normal cholesterol levels. It is becoming more and more apparent that homocysteine levels as well as inflammation levels are a far better marker in predicting future heart disease.

A folic acid deficiency can result in many additional non-heart related health problems as well—both mental and physical. Folate deficiencies can result in depression. Studies have shown that folate helps the brain to produce S-adenosyl-methionine (SAM-e), which has significant antidepressant effects. Folate is a necessary component in our body's ability to manufacture SAM-e. This may well be a key in explaining the observation that depressed people have more cardiac events.

Folate has also been shown to help mitigate liver damage in patients taking the drug, Methotrexate for rheumatoid arthritis.

If you are one of those with high homocysteine and folic acid supplementation has not helped in reducing your homocysteine levels, there is a blood test that can be obtained to determine exactly how much folic acid your body is assimilating. The test is not widely used and is known as a "neutrophilic hypersegmentation index." It measures the amount of folate your system is utilizing. For those who cannot find a place to obtain the test, your doctor can draw your blood and send it to Meridian Valley Labs (425-271-8689). (www.meridianvalleylab.com).

SUNGLASSES: PROTECT YOUR EYES

We have been pretty much aware of how overexposure to the sun can affect our skin; however, there is another overexposure that is even more dangerous if not addressed. That overexposure pertains to our eyes and how the sun's rays can affect eyes. Without the sun we wouldn't exist. We enjoy the light benefits, warmth and vitamin D, however, many of us fail to take appropriate steps to protect our eyes, as well as our skin. Generally speaking, our bodies possess the ability to replace and repair blood cells and even tissue. What cannot be replaced are the cells of the lenses of the eyes so it is imperative that we adequately protect them. We should have appropriate sunglasses while enjoying the outdoors.

The retinas of our eyes contain a marvelous workhorse known as the macula. Because the macula works so hard, it needs adequate nutritional fuel as well as protection from extraneous threats such as the sun. Research has shown that when ultra violet-B (UVB) radiation damages the eyes over lengthy periods of time, the ultimate price may end up in conditions such as cataracts, corneal damage or macular degeneration. The word cataract has often been associated with aging eyes, but there's much more to the story. Many cataracts are a direct result of radiation from the sun according to available literature on protecting vision. For this reason, we need to begin protecting our eyes at an early age, keeping in mind the fact that nutrition for the eyes is also essential and specific. According to alternative physicians 6 mg. of lutein, zeaxanthins, bilberry, quercetin, L-Taurine, zinc, vitamins A & D, as well as N-acetyl Cysteine in adequate amounts will be found in good vision-directed supplements.

Years ago, sunglasses consisted of dark glass with a dark coating for convenience. These older sunglasses actually caused the pupils of the eyes to become open and enlarged in response to the darkness. Once the pupils were opened the sun's UV rays would be able to damage the opened pupils. The darkened glass provided no protection. Today, many sunglasses are treated chemically or coated to protect from UV rays, but we must take steps to assure that the sunglasses we are wearing provide us with as close to 100 percent protection from the sun's rays, as possible. Sunglasses that state they provide absorption up to 400 nanometers basically are indicating they provide 100 percent blockage of UV rays. Dark tints are no assurance of screening protection. The glasses must be labeled with UV protection information. Part of that label should state that the glasses provide at least 90 percent UV protection or even better, 100 percent protection. They should also screen out 75 to 90 percent of visible light, based on recent medical literature. There are many types of glasses that provide differing functions. Polarizing merely means they cut reflective glare of beaches, water and help while driving; although today, most polarizing glasses also protect from UV rays, but you must check to be certain.

Additional information was provided by other organizations suggesting that wide-brimmed hats be used to provide even more light protection. Children's eyes require the same early protection according to the literature. Research indicates that people with light colored eyes; blue, green, and hazel are more susceptible to eye damage from the sun. Any person with existing eye damage must also protect the eyes for every moment while out in the sun or daylight.

For more information on UV protection, call Prevent Blindness America, a volunteer organization at 1-800-331-2020.

SYNDROME X—"INSULIN RESISTANCE" MORE PREVALENT THAN ONCE BELIEVED

The results of your blood tests indicates your LDL "bad" cholesterol is high and your HDL "good" cholesterol is low. The doctor than informs you that your triglycerides are also high. You tend to like carbs and sweets. You may even show signs of low blood sugar (hypoglycemia). You are a little overweight or perhaps obese and the doctor isn't too thrilled about the state of your blood pressure. It's a bit too high and normal conventional protocol subscribes to the theory that you have a deficiency of statin drugs and blood pressure medications.

These symptoms along with fatigue, anxiety and other unexplained "out of sorts" feelings may well be indicators of another pre-diabetic condition most doctors fail to diagnose. The condition is now called "Syndrome X" or "insulin resistance."

According to Dr. Jonathan Wright, he refuses to prescribe any medications until he has obtained a blood test known as glucose tolerance, insulin resistance test. Many physicians merely prescribe the glucose tolerance (GT) aspect of the test and never go the extra step to determine if the patient may have insulin resistance, according to Wright. He states this condition is very often totally undiagnosed and treated.

Insulin resistance means that your pancreas works especially hard when you eat or drink refined sugars, high fructose corn syrup, dextrose or sucrose. Yet, your regular blood sugar test may show up normal. The pancreas produces large quantities of insulin to clear the blood stream. However, if a patient is predisposed to insulin resistance, cells that receive insulin become resistant to the repeated exposures to sugar and the pancreas is now working double duty, according to Dr. Wright. He explains that insulin resistance can cause the kidneys to retain sodium, LDL cholesterol may become high and HDL may be low. The adrenals produce too much adrenaline; hence, the blood pressure increases.

Dr. Wright states that addressing high cholesterol and high blood pressure with drugs prior to running the GT-IRT is tantamount in many cases, to attempting to place a lid on a pot of boiling water to stop it from overflowing. He is opposed to merely treating symptoms. Wright states that all cases of type 2 diabetes were first cases of insulin resistance, most likely for many years before turning into actual type 2 diabetes. The disorder also puts patients at greater risk for heart disease according to a report in "Arteriosclerosis, Thrombosis, and Vascular Biology," August 2001.

Dr. Wright explained that quite frequently patients entering his clinic have been shown to have insulin resistance that was never diagnosed. His treatment? He instructs patients to eliminate refined sugar, high fructose corn syrup and enriched breads and flour from their diets. It's not easy because for the past 50 years, we have become a nation of chocoholics and sugar addicts. He suggests that in order to avoid insulin resistance as well as treating the disorder, we shop the outer perimeter of the grocery store. Get fresh vegetables, whole fruits and meats. Dr. Wright believes that a higher protein and lower carbohydrate diet will help to keep blood sugar levels balanced. Regular exercise is essential to defeating this disorder. He also places his patients on vitamins and specific supplements. These three protocols, he says, will address both cholesterol and blood pressure, if indeed the culprit is Syndrome X (insulin resistance). Wright believes that by addressing the source of the problem through diet, exercise and supplementation, patent medications can be avoided. Wright says that type 2 diabetes is a "burgeoning epidemic," mostly because the pre-condition is not addressed.

Wright also states that while there are other causes of high blood pressure, high cholesterol and triglycerides, he always attempts to rule out insulin resistance before attempting to prescribe medications.

He suggests you ask yourself these questions: Do you have hypoglycemia? Does anyone in your family have type 2 diabetes? Do you consume refined sugars and carbohydrates? Are your cholesterol or triglycerides high? Is your blood pressure high? If so, you may want to ask your physician to rule out insulin resistance by obtaining the GT-IRT. Dr. Wright states that by following his strategies of eliminating refined sugars and carbs, along with exercise and supplementation, you can greatly decrease your chances of ending up with type 2 diabetes. Even more, you will enjoy life much more!

Dr. Wright suggests there are good combinations of specific supplements to assist treating this disorder available at reputable heath food stores or at his Tahoma Clinic. (425) 264-0059.

THYROID—TSH RANGES HAVE BEEN CHANGED—YOUR OLD TEST MAY MEAN SOMETHING DIFFERENT TODAY

We have all either known someone or have experienced the situation ourselves. We complain of symptoms. The doctor orders tests. The tests all come back normal and he/she informs us that we are just fine because the test results fell into the "normal" range. Most doctors don't outwardly express it, but many think it's all in your head. They sometimes use the old term "neurasthenia" to make you feel less like a hypochondriac. Fact is, neurasthenia, means they believe "it's all in your head."

It may not be "all in your head" based on recent revisions to some of those "normal" blood test range guidelines. A major change has occurred in the revision of the numbers used to detect acceptable thyroid function. One newly revised test, known as thyroid-stimulating hormone (TSH) may indicate that millions of us with various symptoms could well have abnormal thyroid function, according to the American Association of Clinical Endocrinologist (AACE).

TSH is a hormone produced by the pituitary gland to stimulate the production of thyroid hormone. Past guidelines determined that TSH levels ranging from 0.5 to 5.0 were considered normal. New guidelines narrow that range from 0.3 to 3.04, an almost 2 full point difference. Many alternative physicians believe that even a figure of 3.04 is too high. They suspect that commencement of thyroid disease begins at any level over 2.0. Alternative physician, Dr. Joseph Mercola, likes to see TSH levels at 1.5 or lower.

Why is the thyroid so important? This little butterfly-like gland lying beneath the Adam's apple has more importance to your well-being than you may realize. Hormones produced by the thyroid gland influence almost every organ, tissue and cell in the body. Undiagnosed and untreated hypothyroidism (under active thyroid) can lead to muscle weakness, osteoporosis, depression, heart disease and high cholesterol according to the AACE.

The new guidelines should help those who were symptomatic but told their thyroids were within the then "normal" ranges. These are people who had no explanation for their fatigue, depression, weight gain, anxiety, forgetfulness, constipation, feeling too hot or too cold, felt heart rate disturbances and suffered unexplained hair loss. This is not to suggest that every case of depression, weight gain, fatigue or other listed symptoms assures one is suffering from an under-active thyroid. This segment on the thyroid is merely meant to provoke interest in those who have been lost in the shuffle. It is meant to encourage them to conduct some homework in getting to the bottom of their health problems. These patients may wish to re-consult their physicians about the new guidelines and the possibility they may have an under-active thyroid in need of attention. The doctor may also take additional thyroid tests to obtain a more thorough picture.

Who is at risk?

According to the AACE, women are the major victims of under active thyroid, especially women who have recently given birth. In fact, women are five to eight times more likely to be diagnosed with thyroid disorders than men. It is also recommended that menopausal women be tested for TSH levels, especially those suffering hot flashes and mood swings. The elderly are also subject to changes in thyroid function and should also be tested.

There are surprising substances that can interfere with thyroid function, such as soy, and foods in the broccoli, cabbage, cauliflower family. They can inhibit iodine absorption in some patients. That does not mean one should avoid such good foods. One with thyroid difficulties should be aware of such problems

Alternative physicians like Dr. Mercola, were years ahead of their time in recognizing and addressing the guidelines. Many other alternative physicians are highly suspicious of any TSH levels over 2.0, especially when accompanied by symptoms of hypothyroidism. They feel that by catching the levels prior to reaching 3.0, they can better control and correct thyroid function. Among the other thyroid tests are the T3 and T4, which is what the synthetic hormone Synthroid is made of. Alternative physicians believe these tests must be run as "free" T3 and "free" T4. Unless run as "free" they may not provide adequate data for assessing thyroid function.

One of the more dangerous aspects of a thyroid deficiency is highly elevated "bad cholesterol" level known as low-density lipoprotein (LDL). High cholesterol is one marker alternative physicians use to signal the possibility of under active thyroid.

What affects thyroid levels:

Dr. Andrew Weil explains that eating small amounts of soy may be fine, but advises against supplementing with soy in pill form or attempting to eat an over abundance of soy products. One of the problems, according to Mary Shomon, author of *Living Well With Hypothyroidism* is that soy is known to be a goitrogen—substance that depress thyroid function, especially if one has existing thyroid disease. Shomon says, "Isoflavones, the key components of soy that make them so potent as a possible substitute for hormone replacement, mean that soy products, while touted as foods and nutritional products—often are used and act as like a hormonal drug. If you have a diagnosed or undiagnosed thyroid problem, or a history of autoimmune disease, over-consumption of soy isoflavones can potentially trigger a thyroid condition." It is also interesting to note that two of the Food & Drug Administration's (FDA) own researchers have objected to the FDA's approval of the health claims regarding soy products.

Alternative physicians state that fluoride is another antagonist of iodine. Additionally, researcher, Ray Peat, Ph.D. explains that the wrong kinds of fats such as polyunsaturated fats, trans-fats interfere with thyroid function as well. He recommends extra-virgin olive oil and coconut oil.

Test yourself—

Dr. David Williams and Dr. Robert Rowen both suggest an easy home test to get an idea of your iodine levels. They suggest you dab your stomach or other fatty area with iodine about the size of a quarter. If the iodine disappears within several hours, it may mean your levels are too low. If it remains for eight to 24 hours, you most likely have adequate iodine. It is important not to ingest any pharmaceutical iodine.

Another home thyroid test suggested by Dr. David Williams and Dr. Robert Rowen is a technique wherein patients measure their temperature immediately upon awakening in the morning. Place a basal thermometer in the armpit, try not to move for about 10 minutes and if your temperature is lower than 97.8 for 10 days straight, they believe you may have what is termed subclinical hypothyroidism. Alternative physicians suggest the use of Armour thyroid if there is evidence of an under active thyroid because it encompasses the entire spectrum of thyroid hormones. They believe Synthroid, the pharmaceutical used by conventional physicians, may not be adequate because it is limited to one hormone, T4.

There are two books for those who may think they have symptoms of hypothyroidism or have already been diagnosed with hypothyroidism. They are, *The Thyroid Solution*, by Ridha Arem, M.D. and *Living Well with Hypothyroidism* by Mary Shomon.

Considering the changes in guidelines, it would be a good idea to ask your doctor to look a little further if you feel you are displaying symptoms.

Iodine and Iodide for thyroid

Most of us know iodine as that red burning liquid our parents put on our early childhood wounds. I remember the bottle had skull and crossbones on it to indicate it was highly poisonous. However, it appears that another form of digestible iodine is much more important to our health.

Iodine is essential to thyroid function and the thyroid gland influences most all of our organs, tissue and cells. For that reason, we want to do what we can to assure the organ is "fed" properly with enough iodine to make it function well.

Dr. Jonathan Wright believes we are consuming far too little iodine on a daily basis. He also feels the American Recommended Daily Allowance (RDA) for iodine is far too low. Wright refers to researcher physician and endocrinologist, Dr. Guy Abraham who has conducted numerous studies and has published many articles on thyroid function and iodine since 2002. Dr. Abraham says that adequate intake of iodine could help reduce many American maladies from breast to prostate cancers. He points to the American RDA (150 mcg.) for iodine as being far less than that of the average intake of the Japanese (13.8 mg.). The Japanese obtain their iodine largely through seaweed and seaweed products. Abraham notes both breast and prostate cancers in Japan are among the lowest in the world. Japan is a nation with one of the lowest iodine deficiencies in the world as well.

There are many types of iodine, some are considered dangerous and even pre-cancerous, according to Abraham, Wright and most alternative physicians. Alternative physicians consider radioactive iodine used for purposes of testing to be one of the least desirable and most dangerous.

Dr. Abraham also points out that both iodine and iodide are needed for overall good health. The manner in which both iodine and Iodide were absorbed and which parts of the body utilized both, determined his decision that both were needed.

One rather interesting observation of Dr. Abraham's was that a simple form of iodine and iodide used to treat iodine deficiency in the 1920's (Lugol's Solution) was replaced by the manmade types of iodine after World War II. He stated that this change from the natural to man-made proved to hinder good health and he suggests that iodine deficiency be treated naturally as it was pre-World War II. It can be obtained only by prescription and such treatment should be adopted under a doctor's care.

Both Dr. Abraham and Dr. Jonathan Wright also point out that during the course of their particular iodine treatment studies, measurements of iodine were taken through 24-hour urine samples to test the efficacy of the iodine treatment and absorption. Almost immediately during the course of these urine samplings, Abraham noted various toxic metals (lead, mercury) were also found in the urine. This indicated the supplementation was removing these dangerous elements from the system, according to Abraham. Additionally, after months of treatment, fluoride and bromide as well as aluminum were excreted in the urine.

Many American diets operate on a "taste" basis and we eat what we have a "taste" for which oftentimes results in poor nutrition including inadequate intake of iodine. When was the last time you ate a seaweed product? I confess, me too.

At any rate, there is so much to learn about the proper forms of iodine and iodide that are available. It is important also to understand we can take too much. If we have low iodine levels, unfermented soy products can pose a problem in that unfermented soy can inhibit iodine absorption. Certain other foods such as turnips, cabbages and cauliflower are considered goitrogens and can inhibit iodine absorption. There are also certain people who have iodine allergies and for that reason, any increase in iodine consumption should be discussed with a physician. Dr. Abraham has prepared a pill form known as Idoral. There is also a combination known as Triodide.

Wright lists reference books on thyroid and iodine. ***Iodine: Why you need it, Why You Can't Live Without It***, by David Brownstein, M.D. can be purchased from Medical Alternative press 1-888-647-5616. *Breast Cancer and Iodine* by David Derry, M.D. Ph.D. is also available from Trafford Publishing at 1-888-232-4444.

VIOXX AND OTHER COX 2 INHIBITORS POSE PROBLEMS

There is a lesson we can all learn from the Vioxx hearings. These hearings presented a microcosm of what goes on with medicine today. We have seen a glimpse of the entire drug approval process—as well as its flaws. It seems things at the "Screaming Monkey Research Labs" are not going very well at all. (I saw Homer Simpson drive by that building, so I know it really exists).

Problems arose when somebody began listening to the chorus of mice and decided to blow the whistle on older studies that indicated a certain class of drugs had negatively affected the cardiovascular system of the little critters. Newer studies clearly showed a higher risk of heart attack and stroke among certain people taking Vioxx.

Many patients operate under the misconception that if a drug is unsafe, its harmful effects will quickly be discovered and it will be removed from the marketplace. Not true. The painkiller, Vioxx was approved for children one week prior to being yanked off the shelves on September 30, 2004. I first read reports of problems with Vioxx in 1999 when Dr. Joseph Mercola predicted trouble. In 2001, I once again read additional warnings in the newsletter "Worst Pills/Best Pills." Vioxx is from a class of drugs known as Cox 2 inhibitors. People need to be informed when problems arise with medications and they should be made aware publicly as soon as the problems surface.

As you can see, the disclosure of issues with Vioxx, has been a long time in the coming and who knows how many have been affected as a result of being unaware of the problems with Cox 2 inhibitors. Research has shown that this class of drugs can create conditions that may potentially cause harm to the cardiovascular system.

Cox 1 and Cox 2 work together

Early studies on mice found that by selectively blocking the cardio-protective Cox 2 enzyme, while leaving the Cox 1 enzyme intact, an imbalance occurs creating an environment that may promote both blood clotting and blood vessel constriction. According to *Science Magazine*, The Cox 1 enzyme creates thromboxane A2 that can cause platelet aggregation (clotting, stickiness) and Cox 2 enzymes are the major source of prostacyclin, a protein that counters the effects of Cox 1 enzymes by promoting blood vessel dilation and inhibiting platelet aggregation.

So what do you suppose happens when Cox 2 enzymes are isolated and blocked? It is believed this may be allowing the Cox 1 to go unchallenged; hence, an environment conducive to blood clotting may exist.

In the November 2004 issue of *"Worst Pills/Best Pills,"* formerly unpublished data obtained through litigation, indicate Bextra, another Cox 2 inhibitor, was found to have created the similar adverse events as Vioxx. The study further showed actual effectiveness of Bextra to be comparable to Ibuprofen, Naproxen and Diclofenac, which were used in the same trials.

In defense of the pharmaceuticals, it was their own recent studies that disclosed the higher rate of heart attack among users of Vioxx. It's just too bad they hadn't noticed when the initial studies had been conducted.

As Food and Drug Administration (FDA) scientist, David Graham, M.D., stated to lawmakers, several other drugs should be closely watched as well as the Cox 2 inhibitors.

He spoke of Crestor, a strong statin drug that can potentially create muscle breakdown, especially for those over age 65 and those with low-thyroid conditions; Meridia, a diet-medication that has created rapid heart beat and high blood pressure in some; Bextra, which created increased heart attack risks in those with heart disease and arthritis; Accutane, an acne medication that may create birth defects; Serevent, a drug used to treat asthma, has a small risk of exacerbating the asthma and in a few cases, believed to have caused death.

Doesn't it bother anyone that pharmaceuticals take a "one size fits all," approach for many medications? Senior citizens are clearly at a higher risk of not processing medications as well as younger people because of metabolic and liver slow-down, yet seniors consume most of our medications. Risk versus benefit is the key and patients should know whether their medication, (Vioxx in this case), is going to cause them to trade in an upset stomach for a heart attack.

WATER: ADEQUATE CONSUMPTION CAN DECREASE RISK OF HEART ATTACK

Water represents cleansing both in a metaphoric sense and in a good health sense. The Bible even associates fountains and water to spiritual cleansing.

Our entire bodies are comprised of about 75% water. Our brains consist largely of good fats and water. It makes sense that adequate pure water intake would be needed to keep our bodies and brains in good working order.

Water can help decrease heart attack

According to Susan M. Kleiner, PhD, University of Washington, "Scientific evidence now shows that water can help prevent heart disease, high blood pressure and other serious health problems." Kleiner writes in the January issue of Bottom Line Health, of one study conducted by doctors at Loma Linda University in California that found people who drink five or more glasses of water a day, actually cut their risk of heart attack in half. (Of course, those with kidney disease or restricted water intake for other medical reasons would not be able to increase water consumption). Another study from Harvard researchers showed that men who drank ll glasses of beverage per day cut their risk of bladder cancer in half over men who drank 6 glasses daily. Those who drank six glasses cut their risks over those who drank only one glass.

Serendipitous discovery

Those more recent "discoveries" were nothing new to Iranian physician, Dr. F. Batmanghelidj, who was imprisoned for 25 months during the reign of The Ayatollah. Dr. F. Batmanghelidj treated thousands of fellow political prisoners in an Iranian hospital; however, the Iranian government would supply no medications with which to treat his patients. Prisoners were given limited food but they had access to abundant supplies of water. Dr. Batmanghelidj had no choice. He had his patients drink lots of water, and found that amazingly, most who drank copious amounts of water were in far better health and had recovered from numerous disorders, both physical and emotional. Dr. Batmanghelidj says he learned that chronic dehydration could be the root cause of many diseases. He also feels that most of us are dehydrated. His book, *Your Body's Many Cries For Water*, was written after his release as a political prisoner.

Dr. Batmanghelidj writes that we are suffering dehydration long before we feel thirsty and that we should establish a regular habit of drinking, at the very least, 8 glasses of pure water daily. He believes that many of our maladies can be treated with pure water, not prescription drugs.

I realize my own experience is anecdotal, but the more pure water I drink, the better I feel. My skin shows it, and I seem to have more energy. It's a task for me to force myself to drink water and only when I set up half-gallon bottles of water, do I consciously make the effort. It's strange that something so simple can seem such a task. We are fortunate to live in a land where we have such access to water whenever we want it. We need to take advantage of the present availability of water for our body's sake.

It might be helpful for those who resolve to diet that they understand a lack of water can actually cause us to have greater appetites. Our body is crying for more water, not food. He also believes lack of pure water can lead to joint pain (tissues require large amounts of water to maintain lubrication, according to Dr. Batmanghelidj). It is helpful when attempting to lose weight, to keep our bodies well hydrated.

Dr. Batmanghelidj further asserts that even a slight drop in total body water can cause memory problems and even mild depression. He does not count coffee or sodas as a positive liquid intake in meeting our body's requirements for fluids. He stresses we drink pure water.

His book, along with the other medical findings, are extremely eye-opening and there is no way I can cover everything I've read today, however, I've gleaned enough to understand that increasing our intake of pure water, or filtered water, is certainly worth a try, especially since it's so abundant, inexpensive and there are no negative side-effects. Well, maybe the obvious trips to the lav, but that's a small price to pay.

WHITE TEA AND GREEN TEA ARE SUPERIOR FOR HEALTH

White tea

Just as modern medical science has come around to "discovering" that green tea has numerous health benefits, a new tea is quickly moving up to prove even more healthful. It only took about 25 years for the conventional medical community to acknowledge the benefits of green tea so how long do you suspect it will take them to "discover" the amazing benefits of white tea? White tea has at least double the antioxidant punch as green tea. White tea is a less processed much more delicate tasting tea than green tea. It is created by picking the early spring buds which give it a much more delicate taste than green tea. Less processing means stronger antioxidant properties are contained within the tea. Don't get me wrong; green tea is an excellent antioxidant. It's a tremendous step in the right direction especially when it replaces sodas and sugary drinks, but white tea appears to be far superior.

One study indicates white tea extract (WTE) is not only a better multi-tasking preparation with more antioxidant power than green tea, but it may also be possess anti-viral and anti-bacterial properties. In addition it may possess anti-fungal qualities that retard fungal growth. Its use may be applicable for prophylactic application against bacteria, especially staphylococcus and streptococcus, two treacherous culprits.

Studies conducted at Pace University, and presented at the May 2004 meeting of the American Society for Microbiology, "suggest that white tea extract may have an anti-viral effect on human pathogenic viruses." The Pace studies also indicated that WTE has an anti-fungal effect on penicillium chrysogenum and Saccharomyces cerevisiae. The study states, "In the presence of WTE, Penicillium spores and Saccharomyces cerevisiae yeast cells were totally inactivated. It is suggested that WTE may have an anti-fungal effect on pathogenic fungi."

According to Milton Schiffenbauer, Ph.D., a microbiologist and professor in the Dept. of Biology at Pace University's Dyson College of Arts and Sciences, "Past studies have shown that green tea stimulates the immune system to fight disease," He states, "Our research shows White Tea Extract can actually destroy in vitro the organisms that cause disease. Study after study with tea extract proves that it has many healing properties. This is not an old wives tale, it's a fact."

The study basically indicates white tea is better than green tea for its possession of anti-viral an anti-bacterial qualities. During the course of the study, toothpastes such as Aim, Aqua fresh, Colgate, Crest and Orajel showed anti-bacterial and anti-viral enhancement with the addition of white tea extract. White tea extract exhibited an anti-fungal effect on Penicillium chrysogenum and Saccharomyces cerevisiae.

According to Milton Schiffenbauer, "White tea extract may have application in the inactivation of pathogenic human microbes, i.e., bacteria, viruses, and fungi." Additionally, in very preliminary studies, researchers at the Linus Pauling Institute have found that white tea appears to have an ability to inhibit mutations in bacteria. The small studies with rats showed the tea-inhibited mutagenicity in DNA damaged cells of rats.

The research is ongoing but I doubt there is a question as to whether a cup of green tea or white tea is better for anyone than that glass of highly acidic soda that contains 10 spoons of sugar or the questionable substance, aspartame.

Green tea

A 1999 study in the American Journal of Clinical Nutrition, found that study participants drinking green tea, burned calories at a faster rate than those using straight caffeine or placebos. That's good news. But other studies have found even more reason to drink up.

Green tea, White tea fight cancer/heart disease

Green tea has many components that not only help with weight loss, but also provide protective qualities to every part of our bodies from our skin to our hearts. Some studies have shown that a potent antioxidant in green tea was reported to have killed human cancer cells in laboratory experiments. The ingredient, known as epigallocatechin-3-gallate, (EGCG) was reported by researchers at Case Western Reserve University in Cleveland, as having killed cancer cells in samples of skin, lymph system and prostate tissue from both humans and mice. It did so without harming any healthy cells, according to the researchers.

Other studies indicate that the flavonoids in green tea, and even to a small degree, black tea, helps to lower bad LDL (low-density lipoprotein) cholesterol, and assist in reducing platelet aggregation (the blood sticking that causes clots). It is also believed that polyphenols found in green tea decrease the production of a protein that causes blood vessels to constrict and reduces the flow of oxygen to the heart. (The protein, endothelin-1, is believed to be associated with the development of heart disease). Researchers believe, polyphenols are what make red wine and grapes so helpful in fighting heart disease.

Green tea, White tea and skin cancer

The anti-oxidant power of green tea is what researchers believe helps fight many cancers. The benefits are not limited to internal organs. The ingredients can improve the health of the skin and protect skin from ultraviolet rays both when consumed internally and applied topically.

One of the most apparent discoveries in most all of what I read in reports and studies on these natural substances, is that, in most all cases, what is good for one part of the body, is also good for the entire body. That is in stark contrast to what I read in the Physician's Desk Reference regarding pharmaceuticals, which almost always include warnings of dangers to other organs, most commonly the liver. These warnings include the necessity to conduct regular blood tests for those taking such prescribed medications.

In the preparation of green tea, remember, "Boiled tea, is spoiled tea." Place your teabags into very hot, not boiling, water.

For those of you who are presently on prescribed medications and are considering adding green tea or white tea to your diet, make sure to clear it first with your doctor. Also, note that all of the benefits of green tea are found in white tea as well.

NOTE: I have also read reports that green tea contains fluoride and that should be taken into account when assessing the total consumption of such teas.

Resources

Prescriptions for Healthy Living
Dr. James Balch
800-728-2288
770-399 5617

Health Alert
Dr. Bruce West
5 Harris Court N6
Monterey, Cal 93940-57d53
831-372-2103

Health Science Institute
819 N. Charles St.
Baltimore, MD 21201.
203-699-4416

Alternatives
Dr. David Williams
800-219-8591
drdavidwilliams.com

Nutrition & Healing
Dr. Jonathan V. Wright
819 N. Charles St.
Baltimore, Md. 21201
203-699 3683

Stephen Sinatra, M.D.
New England Heart &
Longevity Center
800-784-0863
Drsinatra.com

Julian Whitaker, M.D.
Health & Healing
888-886-8213

Robert Jay Rowen, M.D.
Second Opinion
P.O. Box 467939
Atlanta, Ga 31146-7939
800-728-2288
770-339-5617

Worst Pills/Best Pills
Public Citizen
1600 20th St. N.W.
Washington, DC 20009
www.worstpills.org

Dr. Joseph Mercola
Optimal Wellness Center
1443 W. Schaumburg
Suite 250
Schaumburg, IL 60194
847-985-1777
Mercola.com

Susan Lark, M.D.
7811 Montrose Raod
Potomac, Md 20854
Drlark.com
877-437-5275

Health Alert
Dr. Bruce West
5 Harris Court, N6
Monterey, Ca 93940-5753
831-372-2103

Center for Integrative Medicine
Burton Berkson, M.D.
741 N. Alamda Blvd
Las Cruces, N.M. 88005
505-524-3720

Nan Kathryn Fuchs, PhD
P.O. Box 467939
Atlanta, Ga 31146
800-728-2288

Marcus Laux, N.D.
Naturally Well Today
P.O. Box 2040
Forrester Center, WV 25438
800-264-4871

Index

978-0-595-38162-3
0-595-38162-6